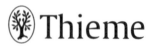

Essays in Medical Ethics

Plea for a Medicine of Prudence

Giovanni Maio, MD
Physician
Philosopher
Chair of Medical Ethics
Director of the Institute of Medical Ethics and History of Medicine
University of Freiburg
Freiburg, Germany

Thieme
Stuttgart · New York · Delhi · Rio de Janerio

Library of Congress Cataloging-in-Publication Data is available from the publisher

Important note: Medicine is an ever-changing science undergoing continual development. Research and clinical experience are continually expanding our knowledge, in particular our knowledge of proper treatment and drug therapy. Insofar as this book mentions any dosage or application, readers may rest assured that the authors, editors, and publishers have made every effort to ensure that such references are in accordance with **the state of knowledge at the time of production of the book.**

Nevertheless, this does not involve, imply, or express any guarantee or responsibility on the part of the publishers in respect to any dosage instructions and forms of applications stated in the book. **Every user is requested to examine carefully** the manufacturers' leaflets accompanying each drug and to check, if necessary in consultation with a physician or specialist, whether the dosage schedules mentioned therein or the contraindications stated by the manufacturers differ from the statements made in the present book. Such examination is particularly important with drugs that are either rarely used or have been newly released on the market. Every dosage schedule or every form of application used is entirely at the user's own risk and responsibility. The authors and publishers request every user to report to the publishers any discrepancies or inaccuracies noticed. If errors in this work are found after publication, errata will be posted at www.thieme.com on the product description page.

Some of the product names, patents, and registered designs referred to in this book are in fact registered trademarks or proprietary names even though specific reference to this fact is not always made in the text. Therefore, the appearance of a name without designation as proprietary is not to be construed as a representation by the publisher that it is in the public domain.

© 2017 by Georg Thieme Verlag KG

Thieme Publishers Stuttgart
Rüdigerstrasse 14, 70469 Stuttgart, Germany
+49 [0]711 8931 421, customerservice@thieme.de

Thieme Publishers New York
333 Seventh Avenue, New York, NY 10001 USA
+1 800 782 3488, customerservice@thieme.com

Thieme Publishers Delhi
A-12, Second Floor, Sector-2, Noida-201301
Uttar Pradesh, India
+91 120 45 566 00, customerservice@thieme.in

Thieme Publishers Rio de Janeiro,
Thieme Publicações Ltda.
Edifício Rodolpho de Paoli, 25º andar
Av. Nilo Peçanha, 50 – Sala 2508
Rio de Janeiro 20020-906 Brasil
+55 21 3172 2297 / +55 21 3172 1896

Cover design: Thieme Publishing Group
Typesetting by DiTech Process Solutions, India

Printed in Germany by CPI Books GmbH 5 4 3 2 1

ISBN 978-3-13-241136-4

Also available as an e-book:
eISBN 978-3-13-241145-6

FSC
www.fsc.org
100%
Paper from well-managed forests
FSC® C124385

Contents

About the Author

Giovanni Maio is the chair of medical ethics at the Albert Ludwig University of Freiburg, where he heads his own institute. He is both a philosopher and a physician with many years of clinical experience. Maio criticizes the promises of feasibility of an engineered medicine and advocates an ethics of prudence: "We cannot become happy without an insight into the limits of what is feasible and the acceptance of the world as it is."

Introduction

"Everything cannot be everything."

(Ingeborg Bachmann)

Who would want to give up the opportunities that modern medicine offers us today? We owe a lot to them, from the very beginning of our life until its end. Indeed, advances in medicine are the major reason why many of us are alive at all and have not had to die of disease or in an accident. Medicine helps us to live our lives in a more unburdened manner. It saves us when we contract a disease that only a hundred years ago would have been a death sentence. To this extent, it is great achievement that modern, well-functioning medicine is available to us. And yet it is precisely this great and indisputable success that bears the seeds of skewed development of other aspects of modern medicine.

What do I mean by this? By skewed development, I mean the observation that medicine, giddy with its success, secretly promises to have everything under control. It increasingly suggests that today, in the age of highly effective modern medicine, one no longer needs to put up with anything. Cutting edge technologies have made it possible to vanquish diseases, extend life, make the body more beautiful, and permanently cure those suffering from hitherto incurable diseases. But does this mean it can really do everything? In the can-do euphoria trumpeted by many areas of medicine, we are increasingly forgetting one thing. Despite all technology, one aspect of being human is that we lack the ability to determine everything ourselves and that the essential things are not in our hands. A consequence of this "forgetting" is that we are increasingly failing to learn how to cope with this finiteness of our ability. The gap between the exaggerated promises of technology and our inability to deal constructively with limits is in no small measure responsible for great moral dilemmas as well as a growing discomfort with "medicine" that is becoming increasingly dominant in our society.

I have not written this book with the intention of joining the ranks of those "critics of medicine" who use this dissatisfaction in society as an excuse for muckraking. Instead, I would like to draw our attention back to the things that humans do not and can never really have under control despite all our technological capabilities. I would like to speak about the limits of what is feasible. Rather than complaining that humans cannot shape everything themselves, I will argue that it may even be good that the essential things remain beyond the grasp of engineering.

Sensitivity to Limits

The increasingly disturbing imbalance in modern medicine demands that we reflect on and question the basic premises of our current approach to the world. This questioning becomes all the more necessary as medicine tends to concentrate only on scientific facts when it deals with human beings. If, in the thinking of large parts of medicine, humans essentially represent only what can be described in scientific terms, then this almost inevitably leads to the attitude that this scientifically describable entity can be changed, manipulated, and transformed. Modern medicine concentrates on changing the external parameters while increasingly losing the ability to distinguish between what must be changed and what one can only react to with the acceptance of something given. Medicine develops entire arsenals for combating disease but offers no guidance in how to deal with and accept what is.

The more we concentrate on doing, the more we lose sight of what lies in front of us, of how important limited entities are for our orientation, and for shaping our lives. Man can only act or produce within the framework of what is given; he does not have absolute freedom to choose this framework. Yet, at the same time, we ourselves are less the result of our own action than an "event" on the substrate of immutable determinants. Modern medicine in particular has long since taken leave of this fundamental insight. The given framework, that which is not doable, that which simply exists—these are concepts that have no place in a medicine oriented toward functionality, programmability, controllability, and efficiency. Just how problematic it can be to banish these fundamental insights is what I would like to demonstrate in this book, which is expressly intended to be an "ethical" book.

Ethics—as a Guide to a Good Life

When we hear the word "ethics" today, we immediately think of the wagging finger, of prohibitions, of restrictions. And when one picks up a book with a title such as this one, one could easily imagine it to be another wagging finger defining limits, demanding we forgo things, and curtailing our options. Yet this is a false understanding of ethics. Since ancient times, the primary purpose of ethical thinking has been to help people lead a fulfilled life. Ethical thinking is thus a guide to a good life. And that is exactly what this book is about.

> The following chapters are not about condemnations, prohibitions, and curtailments. On the contrary, they explore the question of how our life can become "fuller." How can we lead a fulfilled life?

The media often give us very clear messages and very clear-cut solutions. Yet the problems that arise with respect to modern medicine in particular cannot be broken down into shallow messages. Let us look at the limit. It is easy to say that man does not need limits today because he is engaged and should therefore be able to choose everything himself. That sounds good: everyone may choose for himself! Indeed, this expresses the spirit of life in our age, and it was sociologist and philosopher Zygmunt Baumann who expressed this credo in this succinct manner:

> "Postmodern is the exciting freedom to pursue any arbitrary goal and the confusing uncertainty about which goals are worth being pursued."

We already see here that merely by eliminating all limits we do not automatically come any closer to happiness. This is because happiness does not primarily have to do with feasibility, with the means of our dominion over the world, but with knowing something about the where to and why. Where do we want to go, why do we live, what is important in life, what really matters? These are the central questions that ultimately say something about human happiness. When we lose sight of this goal and simply do everything that is possible, then we subject ourselves to the dictatorship of feasibility. Awash in possibilities, we lose the sense of what is essential, namely the question of who we really are and want to be. If we could do everything and wanted everything we could do, we would be nobody. We can only develop an identity when faced with something we cannot do. Identity arises from and is shaped by the limit, the limit of what is feasible but also the limit of what we can wish for.

The Limit as a Requirement for Bounty

In our age, we simply cannot tolerate the presence of a limit. What we really want is to do away with all limits, be able to do everything, decide everything ourselves, have everything the way we want it. But this is a false understanding of freedom and at the same time a false understanding of a good life. Just as the riverbanks make a river possible, limits are also necessary for a human being to comprehend himself as human. Limits must not be understood as a curtailment and restriction but as the requirement for bounty.

Yet what is a valuable limit that creates identity and where does the limitation represent a barrier to be overcome? Examining this question is the challenge of our age. And not only of our age: every epoch must confront the limit in a prudent manner. And when I speak here of prudence, I do not mean it in the sense of rumination that can paralyze us but in the sense of a reflective attitude that can stimulate us to new deeds. To deeds that do not simply spring from the automatic reaction to oppose all limits, but arise as a reflective decision to accept this limit and not another one as a challenge to be overcome. Learning to distinguish between the beneficial limit and the adverse one is what really matters if we want to learn how to deal appropriately with the new possibilities of modern medicine, an approach that will help us to achieve a more fulfilled human existence.

Examples: Who has never wished to live longer? Even to live forever? People have dreamed of this since time immemorial. And yet when we give it some thought it becomes clear that it is precisely the limited time that lends sense and depth to our life.

Further: Who has never toyed with the idea of being someone else; being able to select one's appearance, talents, and capabilities oneself? Everyone has such desires. Yet what kind of life would that be if we could select our own endowments ourselves? Is it not precisely the knowledge that we are this way and not another that challenges us to make something of what we are? If we were to choose everything ourselves, what would we then do with our lives? Is it not precisely the challenge of not choosing for ourselves that makes our life interesting because this is the only way that gives us the chance to prove ourselves?

Thus, the limit is not our writing on the wall; in a sense, it is our salvation.

Further: Many people today desire children who meet their own expectations: healthy, pretty, and intelligent children. It is under-standable that people want children who will not have difficulties in life, who do not simply come as they come but whose existence depends on "optimum launch conditions." Yet here too: How can chil-dren be happy if they know they do not exist simply because they are how they are but because their parents have determined how they have to be? Is it not a blessing that children simply exist without us having selected them? That neither they nor we have to justify our existence?

These are but a few examples to show the direction in which I am thinking in this book. What appears at first glance to be a burden reveals itself on closer inspection as an opportunity. How much freedom lies precisely in the knowledge of that which is simply given!

"It is what it is ...." (Erich Fried)

The fundamental thesis of this book may appear paradoxical at first glance for it is this: fulfilled life is possible only if one learns to deal well with the limit. The limit is thus a requirement for bounty. This sounds contradictory. Yet it is based on a profound insight that I would like to pursue in my book: it is not a matter of prescriptions and prohibitions, but a matter of opening up a depth dimension of life.

The physician and theologist Albert Schweitzer once said that the most beautiful way to excite is to inspire mindfulness. And I admit that nothing is more important to me that to engender a contemplative attitude with the chapters that follow, so as to find paths to a fulfilled life not by way of promises but by way of reflection. Paths that are not obviously there to be followed, but paths which everyone must clear for himself step by step, only by reflecting on the depth dimension of the problems to be examined.

Chapter 1
Meeting in the Petri Dish?

How many people wish nothing more fervently than a child but are unable to have one? Technology can help many of them and yet it also creates new problems which one must take into consideration sufficiently early. This chapter examines the question of why technology alone cannot solve the problem of the desire to have children. It poses the question of how couples desiring children can be helped more comprehensively, for these couples are not customers to whom one can offer new technology but human beings who desire holistic care to see them through the crisis. This chapter also explores the meaning of parenthood arising from the meeting of an egg and sperm in a petri dish and the importance of the relationship between children and their parents, which goes far beyond technology.

Reproductive Medicine between Exigency and Engineered Normality

Within only a few decades, the unborn child that a woman once simply expected without being able to influence its coming in any way has become a seemingly programmable and diagnostically testable object. Medicine has made it a goal to no longer accept the fate of undesired childlessness. And this is a good thing. Many people who were once forced to endure the pain of forgoing children can now become parents with the aid of assisted conception. This indisputably represents a great step forward and is a blessing for many. Thus, we can initially regard reproductive medicine as an invention in the service of mankind.

The classic method of assisted conception is in vitro fertilization (IVF). The technique was developed in the 1960s and 1970s by British gynecologist Patrick Steptoe and physiologist Robert Edwards, who in 2010 received the Nobel Prize for it. This method involves bringing together mature eggs and processed sperm in a petri dish where spontaneous fertilization occurs. The embryos that arise in this manner are implanted into the uterus several days later. The starting point for IVF was initially the medical indication of an exigency such as fallopian tube pathology in the woman. Since then, the technology of fulfilling the desire to have children has become a well-established field of medicine, especially in private practices and clinics. In Germany alone, 200,000 couples make use of the assistance of reproductive medicine. Close to 2% of all children born today come into the world as a result of IVF. That makes at least 100,000 children in the last 10 years. Since the birth of Louise Joy Brown, who in 1978 in Oldham near Manchester was the first person to be conceived in vitro ("in a test tube"), over 4 million children worldwide have been brought into the world in this manner. And yet the success rate for the first attempt is only nearly 16%, which by the way is the success rate of psychological consultation.[1] Of 100 couples, 84 remain childless after the first attempt despite every technological method.

But when the media and the glossy brochures of the respective private clinics continually praise reproductive medicine as an unmitigated success story, they ignore all those many couples who remain childless despite technology. Statistically, each couple must have undertaken five or six attempts before they achieve "success," and this success is often never achieved, especially in the case of older women. Most embryos fertilized in a test tube never become implanted in the uterus. Thus, there are many couples who have to try again and again, and still remain childless in the end. These couples are the real losers. This is true not only because technology has not worked for them but also especially because the promises of the technological options have lured them into a dependency on medicine from whose embrace they can only escape with great effort.

Feasibility

Reproductive medicine, which undertakes to intervene in the beginning of human life, is a particularly clear example of why an exclusively technological approach to the problem of undesired childlessness will necessarily remain deficient. Its deficiencies do not stem per se from too little technology, but from too much; more pre-cisely, they stem from the fact that technology suggests a fundamental feasibility. It conveys the impression that whether one will become a mother or father is only up to oneself because technology can supposedly do everything. Thus, the transformation of reproduction into a technological process also creates standards, which for many women are difficult to ignore. Becoming pregnant, so the implied doctrine goes, is something available to any woman. And should she nonetheless remain childless, then only because she did not make a good enough investment, was not well advised, or simply did not try it often enough. The claim to feasibility conveyed in this manner puts many couples in the situation of hardly being able to escape it: their thoughts, desires, and endeavors henceforth follow the dictate of technological options.

The philosopher Hans Jonas (1903–1993) introduced the concept of the technological imperative for this quandary. He described the demand to follow what is technologically feasible at all times and without reservation:

"Always act in such a way that no technological option remains unused!"

This maxim drastically contradicts what Jonas terms "responsibility": the avoidance of inestimable risks and the recognition of limits. It seems as if the promise of technology would at a stroke blot out and render pointless all implicit questions about the moral justifiability of an action, about its psychological acceptability, or simply its reasonableness. Everything seems possible! Many couples enter reproductive clinics with this underlying sense of euphoria, and they are yanked back into reality all the more forcefully when the birth of a child fails to occur. Technology therefore creates a feasibility quagmire which one finds difficult to escape. To better understand the many problems associated with reproductive medicine, we must ask what it means to concentrate solely on propagating technology as the solution to undesired childlessness, which holds an ancient question of humanity.

Casting Aside Limitations

In addition to the reluctance to address the lack of progeny in any other than a technological manner, the technological imperative holds yet another danger: it knows no limit. Technology infiltrates uncharted realms, and it knows no fear of what is new and no respect for what is. It is invariably geared to change and dynamism. Yet with this drive, technology ensures that even within medicine there is no longer any condition that cannot be made to undergo a technical change or improvement. Everything that is could, as the technological imperative suggests, be made even better! But does this also mean that that which is technologically possible should also be done? That it does not reach limits that arise from contexts other than those of feasibility? Formulating limits that are not set by technology appears totally meaningless from a purely technological perspective. Examples of this casting aside of limits in the area of reproduction include becoming a mother at the age of 64, becoming a mother with the aid of the deceased husband's sperm cells, becoming a mother without a biological father by means of semen from an unknown donor, becoming a mother without having to bear the child (by means of a surrogate mother), becoming a mother without having to be the genetic mother oneself (by means of a donated egg), etc.

Note that my intention is not to make a blanket condemnation of these technological options. Rather, I would like to advocate placing them in a larger framework than the one defined by the technological imperative. For, in all the cases mentioned, far more is occurring than a simple triumph of engineering; more layers of the human existence are involved than mere engineering success, which in the first instance means no more or less than exceeding a limit. The problem of the solely technological approach to the malady of undesired childlessness does not lie in the fact that it blocks out large areas of the world of human life in order to reach its goal, the birth of this long-awaited child. With its limit-exceeding character, it also awakens urges that in large measure it cannot satisfy, and it provokes questions for which it provides no answers. All this which is ignored—the pain, the feeling of "failing," the urges, and the exceeding of limits by means of technology—is ignored and indeed even tabooed in the context of a society that increasingly entrusts itself to the technological imperative. Yet, does not all this comprise the great unruly dark side of the baby take home rate, that shortsighted measure used to express the "success" of reproductive medicine? How are we to respond to the destruction of natural limits caused by the use of reproductive medical technologies and methods? Do children have a right to an unequivocal ancestry? What does it really mean for mothers, fathers, and children; indeed for all of us as a society; to view the state of being a mother, a father, and a child purely from the perspective of technological feasibility? Does it not matter at all to us where we come from and whether our genetic parents have even met in real life?

The child made to order, the child as a product, the child as a result of a manufacturing process—these are notions which can indeed represent something of a threat, notions which I would like to examine in a few steps over the next few pages. With the powerful alliance of medicine and technology, we occasionally lose sight of the fact that technology represents not only a method but also a program that is linked to a very specific mindset. In other words, technological methods reflect premises that often remain implicit yet ensure the very success of the method. For example, IVF presupposes that reproduction is a mere technical challenge and that the human relationships involved are of subsidiary importance. What happens on the way between the "desire to have a child" and that child's engineered conception? What concept of human being, what premises are implicit in engineered reproduction? And are these premises really so self-evident?

The Child as a Product: The Logic of Engineering

With respect to engineered reproduction, I regard two aspects of that which I shall call its way of thinking or *internal logic* as particularly important. These are the logic of engineering, which is directed toward a product (the birth of a child), and the logic of depersonalization, which affects the variables of the parenthood this requires, that is, the role of father and mother. While retracing these "logics" may seem a rather dry exercise in light of their gleaming promises, I am convinced that one cannot truly comprehend the particular challenges of modern reproductive medicine if one fails to take this setting into account. Conversely, only the examination of these questions will reveal what a holistic, humane medicine can be and do.[2]

To Manufacture Is to Control

Every naturally conceived child exists because it simply came into the world. Even if its parents wanted it, one cannot say that they had made it or ordered it by engaging in intercourse. On the contrary, the sex act is a necessary condition for the child's existence. Yet the child's existence does not automatically arise from the sexual union of a couple. Whether a child arises from its parents' lovemaking is beyond their control. The philosopher Martin Rhonheimer notes, correctly in my opinion, that no child born can be regarded as the "product of the desire and action of its parents."[3] It is more than that. And precisely because it is more than the product of its parents' desire the child can see itself as given. The child's parents may have planned for it, but the child's actual existence does not come from its parents because it is self-evident that this existence is fundamentally beyond human control.

This recognizance and the knowledge that the child is not made but is something that is simply given could gradually be lost in the technological setting of IVF should we fail to reflect on these dangers soon enough. The engineered arrangement creates the risk of thinking that the artificially conceived person represents the result of an engineering process. One naturally thinks that it is the parents and the doctors who with the aid of technology have caused this person to come into existence. That means that one could be deceived into thinking that this child has not simply come into the world on the basis of immutable determinants but is there only because its parents have used every available means to allow it to arise.

On the contrary, one must remember that IVF is not a process whereby a person comes into existence simply because of technology; rather, that person comes into existence in a manner that despite all technology remains beyond human influence. We run the risk of thinking we ourselves are the motive force in creating human life, and this fundamentally changes our view of the life ostensibly created in this manner. It changes it to the extent that one thinks one has this life under control and is able to bring it about willingly and consciously. Only against the backdrop of this idea does the attitude of *wanting* to bring about this life by any means arise. And only against this backdrop can the technological imperative become a genuine obsession beyond all other contexts.

The danger of this obsession in my eyes is the fundamental problem of the engineered treatment of the desire to have children. One sees it in often unfounded claims of many fertility clinics. For example, the home page of a fertility clinic in Cologne, Germany, states, "Happiness is not happiness without children." At the same time it expresses the promise, "We always make an effort to fulfill your wishes completely." Few will notice that "happiness is not happiness without children" is tantamount to deception and that the promise to "fulfill your wishes completely" is more than misleading in light of the fact over 84% of attempts are initially unsuccessful. It becomes all the more problematic when this engineering mindset combines with denial of the possibility that this desire may never be fulfilled.

The basis of this blind faith in the "success" suggested by reproductive medicine is the attitude of being able to control life. One does not allow life to come of its own accord but degrades it to a product that one can bring about with a specific process arrangement, essentially like any arbitrary object. This tacitly conveyed way of thinking makes us blind to the fact that one simply cannot manufacture human life but can only help it to arise. It is not the making of life that is the basis, rather wanting to serve it, to give it the time and space it needs. This in turn means nothing other than allowing life to be bestowed and not ordered. Is this fundamental insight not becoming increasingly foreign to us under technology's engineering dictate? Luckily, even in the setting of reproductive medicine there are still many parents who actually perceive their child as a gift, especially when they first must experience many unsuccessful attempts. And yet as it necessarily implies an aspect of the immutable, this expression of the gift clashes with the rationality of engineering, which allows no room for the immutable.

Is the Child a Means to an End?

Why is IVF performed? Many reproductive specialists would probably answer, "because they would like to have a child." Accordingly, IVF is the fulfillment of a wish. It is an instrument for making wishes come true. But does this not mean that, without reflection, one also runs the risk of regarding the child to be "produced" by IVF as a means of fulfilling a wish? That one might possibly think that both IVF and its result, the future human being, are good only when there is a need that they address?

The problem that this implies could be expressed as follows. A child whose existence is only meaningful as long as it fulfills a purpose does not possess his own intrinsic meaning and purpose. The child's meaning and purpose are then dependent on the couple's desire to have a child. This also becomes apparent when we put the reproductive specialist's words into the future father's or mother's mouth: "Having a child is good because it fulfills my desire to have a child." We would automatically leave the straight and narrow because we would be making the child an instrument. Moreover, we would not be giving any value to the child's existence *in itself*, as the philosopher Rhonheimer says. Thus, the child would only have value insofar as it fulfills a certain function; it would be an existence *for us*. And the recognition of the child would therefore only be a conditional recognition, not complete and comprehensive as we would all presumably wish for ourselves.

This point reveals a fundamental problem of the engineering approach to the human problem of undesired childlessness. The more imprudently these techniques are applied, the more they can alter our attitudes toward the child and toward undesired childlessness in the long run. Because the increasing use of technology with its promise of feasibility and the all too rare application of holistic care will gradually lead to a situation in which too many people will completely reject the idea that one can only genuinely do justice to a child when one accepts and even embraces from the outset the fact that the desire to have a child will go unfulfilled. Unfulfilled because the child cannot simply be made as the engineered arrangement suggests. What couples should be instructed in is being open to plan B, developing the capability to think in alternatives and not insisting only on the engineered solution. This sensible behavior implies the fundamental attitude that we should always view the desire to have children in a comprehensive context, understanding it as an expression of hope and not as the attitude of being able to do everything ourselves, of having absolutely everything under our own control. What we must preserve despite technology is our inner attitude toward the child, whom we must not approach with the attitude of wanting to place an order. This danger is implicit in modern medicine's strategy of seeking a solely technological solution.

> Every child can be adequately understood only as a gift that is not good because we have desired it for ourselves but because it is good in its own right, and that it is still good even if it had never entered our minds as a "wish."

The more reproductive medicine turns the givenness of human life into a state of being able to order, the more it degrades this life to a means. And that gives rise to an attitude with dire consequences. For when we say that human existence is only good because it has been desired, must we not also accept that there are human existences that (because we have not wished for them) are apparently superfluous and useless and therefore to be regarded as a burden?

It is precisely this transition from life as a gift to life as a means of making wishes come true that we are experiencing in many places today. It is also becoming obvious in the second great range of tasks that modern medicine addresses in connection with the unborn child and which could be characterized as follows. There are many people who have a child but do not know whether they really want it. Moreover, many do not know whether they want *precisely this child* and perhaps not *a different one*, a healthier one, in any case one without disabilities. Thus, in prenatal diagnostics one acts as if it were the most natural thing in the world to immediately reject as unfit a human life that one did not desire in the given form. I will examine this in greater detail in the next chapter. Both branches of modern medicine that concern themselves with the unborn child, engineered reproduction and prenatal diagnostics, share the notion that one can use technology to "make" and "manufacture" human life according to one's own wishes. Life, which in the words of the Lebanese-American author Khalil Gibran (1883–1931) "yearns for itself" and therefore never belongs to us, becomes a product whose characteristics one can specify before it comes into the world. This seems to me to be the fundamental scandal of the logic of engineering in reproductive medicine.

Naturally I do not mean to suggest that everyone involved today thinks this way. Blanket condemnations are not helpful and they do not do justice to people's individual needs, desires, and behavior. In presenting these ideas I would like to show that the increasing use of technology creates a quagmire. Not only does this quagmire make it nearly impossible to avoid using technology, but it also lends plausibility to a certain way of thinking. It is thus a quagmire of thinking that one must resist if one would not like to think in the manner suggested by the technological imperative.

> "Your children are not your children. They are the sons and daughters of the yearning of life for itself. They come through you but not from you, and although they are with you, they do not belong to you. You may give them love but not your thoughts for they have their own thoughts. You may give their bodies a house but not their souls. For their souls live in the house of tomorrow which you cannot visit, not even in your dreams." (Khalil Gibran)

The Child Is Not a Result but a Beginning

The natural conception of a child is ultimately an act of love that is not directed solely toward a certain result. The child may come, but whether or not it will come is not entirely foreseeable and ultimately beyond our reach. Not only is the existence of the child unforeseeable but so are its traits and characteristics. This has given rise to the idea of the gift, to the notion of life is a gift.

Were we now no longer to proceed from "conceiving life" but only from "engineering life," then there would be no more openness, no unpredictability, no more gift. Then the gift would become a product, which in turn would set new standards: not openness but fixedness, not unpredictability but comprehensive technological controllability and programmability, no more hope but the expectation of the product as ordered. If we fully embrace the engineering mindset, we must accept that the result of the production process is determined from the outset. One does not manufacture something blindly; rather, the entire process is geared to the desired product whose characteristics have been determined in advance.

The "born quality" of a person, that is, that which in the opinion of the philosopher Hannah Arendt (1906–1975) causes us to characterize a person as something entirely new that comes into the world, as a genuine *beginning*, shrinks in the logic of engineering to a mere point in a process that technology ostensibly controls and apparently should be controlling increasingly exclusively. Here I would like to expressly emphasize that this loss, this reduction to a product and result, ultimately does not involve the artificially conceived person himself. Everyone, even the embryo floating in a nutrient solution that is screened for suitability and perhaps later rejected, is a life of its own accord and thus a beginning. The one-sidedness encouraged by the logic of engineering applies more to our own perspective and thus to our behavior toward life, including our own. It could cause us to lose sight of the fact that with every person something comes into the world that had not existed before. There is nothing that can cause more astonishment than a new human being if only one would be brave enough to allow and accept him viscerally and intellectually as such a gift.

There is one more aspect that I feel is important: if we understood the child as a product that can be made and not as a beginning in itself, then the child would not only have the right to hold its parents responsible for the state of its existence and possibly accuse them of failing to exercise diligence (in the presence of a disability), it would also have the obligation to thank its parents for production that proceeded "properly." For the first time, the child would not simply be unconditionally present, but as a result of its birth would be burdened with an obligation of gratitude. The engineering mindset not only represents a burden for the parents, who could face action for "negligence." It is also a burden for the children, who owe the fact and manner of their existence to their parents' choice and therefore may not live their lives without feeling the need for reciprocal consideration.

> Practiced imprudently, reproductive medicine imposes a double burden: on future parents the burden of "proper production" and on the children the burden of an obligation of gratitude to their "manufacturers." In both cases, the human being is no longer viewed as a beginning for its own sake.

Just how widespread this thinking has become is evidenced by repeated discussions of late as to whether situations could arise in which a person protests to his parents that they should never have brought him into the world. This thought in itself disturbingly illustrates the extent to which we have already embraced the engineering mindset. We no longer notice what a contradictory issue it is to want to hold one's parents responsible for not having aborted oneself.

When people are no longer conceived but are manufactured in an engineering process, then the "makers" assume a "product warranty" so to speak and are confronted with appropriate claims. From the moment that the most self-evident of self-evident principles—namely that a life is simply present without one being able ask its purpose—is suspended, there can be no more peace and a new human being can no longer arrive without fear. For even if one says yes to this person, one might have done everything wrong.

The Logic of Depersonalization

In addition to the logic of engineering, the transformation of reproduction into a technological process also introduces a second "logic": the logic of depersonalization. It ignores the *relational nature* of reproduction. Indeed, it purposely excludes it. Conception is objectified to the point that the process by which a human being arises appears stripped of any relationship structure. At least we are increasingly less receptive to the notion that the people involved in this technological process that gives rise to a human being are in a human relationship with each other.

Becoming a Father without Personal Relationship. Becoming a Mother without Being Allowed to Be One

This is apparent even with the first IVF process in history, the practice of sperm donation in which not the partner but a third party is involved. This person "donates" sperm for money, in effect selling it as a service. The donor participates in an artificial, that is, mediated, "act of procreation" without entering into any kind of relationship. Neither the woman who will "receive" the sperm knows the one who will "donate" it, nor does the donor know the mother of his future child or even the child itself. And this is intentional! The objectification of the relationship process is even an express condition of this "act." I would in no way like to insinuate that great emotions are not present at the birth of a child conceived in this manner devoid of any relationship. And yet it cannot be denied that a process that originally had its place exclusively within a relationship has become the object of engineered manufacturing. Not only does this ignore that the donation of sperm (i.e., biological fatherhood) cannot really be regarded as a simple service for a fee. It also ignores what it means for the future child thus conceived that it has not arisen from an interpersonal relationship but has only been "produced" using "components" that were not in any human relationship to one another because the sperm and egg came from people who had never met in real life. It is no coincidence that so-called "donor children" complain of having to live with the idea of having arisen in impersonal cold, as Sibylle Steidl has vividly described in several media reports from her perspective of personal involvement.[4] That these children complain of this is due to the taboo that society still places on donating sperm. These complaints illustrate that mankind's fundamental self-image has become unsettled with the advent of the new fertilization methods. This is because no thought has been given to the possibility that humans may have a fundamental need to descend from parents who have a relationship with each other.

We also experience this development towards ignoring the relationship in the case of egg donation, a practice that is still prohibited in Germany. Because it is practiced in many other European countries (such as France, Spain, the Czech Republic, and the Netherlands), many German couples desiring children go abroad. The Viennese cultural and social anthropologist Eva-Maria Knoll has spoken of global "reproductive tourism" in this regard. Here, too, the natural process that gives rise to a human being becomes a purely technological process in which a relationship between the people involved is excluded from the outset. Indeed, the intent is that such relationships remain expressly excluded, for example, the relationship between the egg donor and the child.

> Egg cell donation involves removing hormonally stimulated eggs from a donor, fertilizing them with sperm in vitro, and then implanting them in the recipient's uterus. The child entering the world in this manner is descended from two mothers. It carries the genes of the egg donor, yet was born of the egg recipient, the client. One can refer here to "dissociated" motherhood.

The logic of depersonalization reveals itself as a logic of modularization in connection with sperm donation, more obviously in egg donation, and most explicitly in surrogate motherhood. By this I mean that the entire reproduction process is fragmented, that is broken down into individual components ("modules") that are then recombined. The modularization of reproduction presents us with a new challenge, that of establishing previously unknown familial relationships, especially new family structures in which there is more than one pair of parents.

Origin and Identity

Thus, with third-party sperm donation, one locates a genetic father for one's "own" future child, a father that one knows will never be a part of the child's own world. This represents nothing other than consciously forcing an alien origin on the child, which will invariably become a particular challenge to master. The peculiar feature of this situation is that such alienation from one's own origin, which must be accepted in other cases such as when the father dies early, here is brought about directly and thus in a certain sense demanded. This represents what one could refer to as *willfully bestowing a deficit*.[5] In fortunate cases, this flaw can be managed by appropriately early enlightenment and sensitive treatment of the subject. Yet the question arises as to whether one should follow a path that involves many challenges for the child regardless of the cost.

Sperm donation basically does not involve "dissociated" fatherhood. Here, we have a clear case of third-party fatherhood. The child has only one father from whom it is descended. In the case of egg donation, the child has not only one mother but two mothers from whom it is descended. Not only the egg donor has given the child something essential from herself, namely her genes, the mother bearing the child has also had no small influence on the state of the child's existence. This is not only true because embryo-maternal communication exists, an active exchange between mother and child, but also because the mother by bearing the child influences the child's genes, not by heredity but by epigenetics, by the immediate environment of the maternal organism. For this reason, one can indeed refer to "dissociated" motherhood. And only in this case will the child feel it belongs to both mothers.

Thus, the ethical problems of egg donation concentrate where it is a matter of the identity of the child. With sperm donation, the child is consciously confronted with third-party fatherhood. With egg donation, it is not the third-party egg donor but the duality of one's own descent from two women that poses a challenge. This creates a familial relationship that has never before existed in this form. Until now, the principle *Mater semper certa est!* (The mother is always certain!) has always applied. With egg donation, a child is conceived whose ancestral classification initially had be determined externally because it no longer followed naturally. In Germany, the legal problem has been resolved. There the principle applies that the child "belongs" solely to the mother who gives birth to it. Yet a law was required to define a circumstance that had previously been self-evident. These comments raise the following questions: to what extent can it be advisable to intentionally burden the child and future adult with these great challenges, which can even assume the form of an unreasonable demand? Notwithstanding that a similar experience (for example, in the context of a stroke of fate) could be accepted and possibly even overcome, does that mean that the child should be consciously and deliberately subjected to such an experience?

Social Egg Freezing: Family Planning on Ice

All these problems occur because as it has become transformed into a technological process, human reproduction has also become modularized as if by necessity and because this in turn introduces an arbitrariness into the joining of gametes. This arbitrariness inevitably leads to the next step, the temporal and spatial decoupling of the reproduction process. Social egg freezing represents a particular form of modularization and fractionation of the reproductive process. This somewhat misleading term refers to the freezing of eggs or ovarian tissue for the purpose of using the gametes for a pregnancy at a time of the woman's own choosing.

This freezing represents a method originally intended to remove eggs from young cancer patients to protect them from damage by cancer treatment so they could later be implanted in the event the woman desired children. Whereas this was originally a medically indicated procedure, its intended goal has since changed in that the method is now essentially available on demand. This has given rise to the term social freezing because the indication is contingent upon social factors and not disease. This is about nothing other than establishing a fertilization reserve that one thinks one can fall back on at a time of one's own choosing. This method of storing gametes to create a cache illustrates particularly well the decoupling of reproduction from its biological determinants, here in the form of temporal decoupling.

Just what should we think of this? The method initially appears encouraging. It promises to finally be able to stop the ticking biological clock. It promises nothing less than time. A respected specialist in reproductive medicine was recently quoted in a report in the newspaper *Hamburger Abendblatt* as saying, "With social freezing you gain about ten to fifteen years." The technical terms have hardly been chosen randomly: social freezing suggests that even the ebbing flow of time in the rush hour phase of life is frozen. That makes this method so fantastic because it touches on a human dream, the dream of overcoming time. That at least is the suggestion. But is that really true?

Let us first examine the purely medical aspect. As simple as freezing eggs sounds, the procedure does indeed involve health risks. One egg cell becomes ripe every month. Yet it is necessary to have several eggs for an *in vitro* pregnancy. Therefore, women must first be stimulated with the appropriate hormones. This hormone treatment in itself is not without risks. In any case, it places a burden on the woman as it involves significant side effects such as weight gain, mood swings, and circulatory irregularities. In the worst case, it can result in overstimulation with development of cysts. In addition to the burdens of hormonal stimulation, there are also the burdens of needle aspiration of the eggs. This usually has to be done under general anesthesia and for that reason alone is not without risk. In addition to these considerations, a pregnancy later in life is also associated with higher rates of complication. But there is not only the physical burden but a not insignificant financial burden as well (around 2,000 euros or 2,200 dollars). This does not include the costs of storing the eggs in nitrogen, which run about 300 euros or 330 dollars per year. All these costs are not borne by health insurance funds.

Can We Really Freeze Time?

Even more important is the question of whether this method can really keep the promise of freezing time. From a purely scientific standpoint, it should be noted that female fertility rapidly decreases after the age of 27. If one opts for this method long after the age of 30, then it is really already too late. The numbers support this. The chances of actually becoming pregnant at the age of 35 with a thawed egg that was frozen at age 30 are about 7 to 12%.[6] This means that although the eggs can be preserved as psychological reassurance, this reassurance is in fact rather illusory. Women are thus given a false sense of security. Moreover, this technique promises that a woman can free herself of fate entirely and fully control reproduction. It promises nothing less than greater autonomy. In a recent article in the newspaper *Die Zeit*, a woman referring to social egg freezing was quoted as saying, "Now women themselves can decide how long they want to be able to have children. This means we are no longer at a disadvantage with respect to men."[7] Who does not want to decide themselves how long they can have children? Such a promise is therefore very attractive. Yet, viewed in light of the scientific figures, this promise turns out to be downright deceptive. It may well be that social egg freezing can help a woman over 40 have children. However, there can be no talk of certainty or high probability. In light of figures that hardly inspire confidence, the German Society for Gynecology and Obstetric Medicine has issued an official statement explaining the situation with near-perfect clarity: "The freezing of eggs prior to cancer therapy is justified to allow young cancer patients to become pregnant after the end of therapy. However, the success rates for women over 35 in particular do not represent 'insurance' for using freezing as an instrument of family planning."[8]

This scientific statement contrasts with the public perception of this technique. In any case, there is a gap between the hopes that are still being generated and the official statements of serious scientific societies. Social freezing can also represent a very lucrative commercial exploitation of many women's fears and this shows how damaging the implementation of advertising strategies can be especially in this field. Not only can advertising generate unrealistic hopes, it can also trivialize the risks. Bern gynecologist Michael von Wolff put it very succinctly when he wrote in *Die Schweizerische Ärztezeitung*: "Ultimately only two things are clear: The most reliable way to one's own child is a pregnancy at < 35 years of age and one of the most unreliable is social freezing at > 35 years of age."[9]

Living in Multiple Option Mode

Reproduction is made subject to our desire to control, and the opportunities of reproductive medicine suggest that one could make reproduction fully programmable and available for one's own wishes. Significantly, the web page www.familienleben.ch introduces social freezing with promises such as: "Do children fit into my career plans? Do I first want to enjoy my life without children?" These promises illustrate how close we are coming to forgetting that everything in life has its time. For example, the time for having children is the young period of building and not the older period of being established because only in this way can there be less of an age difference to the child. The technologies suggest it is wrong to subject oneself to the cyclical course of life and to accept it as given. Instead, the individual is given the responsibility for determining the time herself according to her own personal criteria. What initially appears to be a gain could under closer scrutiny turn out to be a handicap. This is because the greatest danger arising from social freezing is its suggestive power.

This method suggests that time can be stopped and one can afford to put off having children. That means that the existence of the technology alone can motivate couples to continually postpone the realization of their desire to have children to a "more suitable" time. Why not? The technology is there. If we consider that we live in an age in which it is ever more difficult for people to make decisions at all, especially decisions affecting one's partner, and if we consider that especially today many people are afraid to commit to one partner because they secretly think there might be better "partner options," then it becomes clear how dangerous this technology is. We live in what Peter Gross has aptly described as a multi-option society. We would like to keep as many options as possible open for as long as possible. We experience every narrowing of our choices as a loss. The moment we decide on a partner, we also decide against many others; thus, we effectively limit our options. In this setting, many people continue to search their entire life for an even better option for their life and miss the opportunity to eventually form a genuine bond. To this extent, technology can become an invitation to remain in this multi-option life and in so doing sacrifice the final opportunity to have a child.

It can be very helpful to consider these very subtle dangers in advance. Consider that the tragic flaw of this technology is that it seduces us to enhance our optional lifestyle even with respect to our progeny and thus to risk walking away empty-handed in the end. This illustrates that there is indeed no connection between broadening the range of options and the freedom to choose one of these options. For we must not forget that the increase in possibilities may well also be accompanied by a lack of freedom, specifically the lack of freedom that results from uncertainty, doubt, hesitation, and fear. Faced with a broad range of possibilities, we become unwilling to risk a decision, fearing that we may make the wrong choice or only the second best and thus fail to achieve the optimum. We now desire to make not only good decisions but also optimal ones in every aspect of life, and this tends to render us unable to make decisions (the article by Claudia Bozzaro[10] in this connection is well worth reading).

This reveals something fundamental: we experience the time pressure of deciding in favor of a family as simply a burden, as a bothersome obstacle. Yet we fail to see that this same biologically determined time pressure can give rise to a value, the value of self-reflection. When we know that we have little time we are forced to reflect on ourselves and to become clear about what life we want to lead. Time pressure can also intensify life because we are forced to seek our identity and ascertain who we want to be. Time pressure is like a magnifying glass that focuses on what is essential. It disciplines us by preventing us from continuing to lose sight of what is important. It urges us to decide now, to make matters clear now, and not to avoid a decision any longer. This means that time pressure can have a cleansing effect as well as a clarifying effect. One can say that time pressure is as painful as it is necessary for a good life. Thus, the great question arises as to whether social freezing actually represents a time gain or whether it really seduces one to avoid taking an unequivocal stand and continuing to shrink from a decision about one's priorities in life.

There is another aspect to be considered. Today, it is very difficult for young women to reconcile their career goals with the goals of having a family in such a way that they can live without conflict. In this setting, having a family is often deferred until it is no longer possible. Now a technology has become available that appears to take the edge off this fundamental problem. Hardly anyone has noticed that here we are resorting to biological means to solve a structural and social problem. Hardly anyone has noticed that we prefer to leave the structural and social factors unchanged in favor of "solving" the problem by placing it squarely on the women's shoulders.

> We prefer to violate the woman's physical integrity than to alter the structural and social circumstances. To my mind, this sharply contradicts the rhetoric of freedom that is employed in implementing social freezing.

Moreover, we isolate the eggs with the assumption that by preserving these cells in a "young" state we have preserved time itself. Far too little consideration is given to the fact that while the eggs are frozen, not only the mother but also her entire environment continues to age during the period of freezing. That means that the gamete may be frozen but not time itself. The woman continues to age. And the woman's environment, her social setting, her habits, all adapt to her advancing age. That means that when one thinks the child could come later because the eggs have been frozen, one must recognize that this child will be born into a comparatively "old" environment. This in turn means that the age difference between the child and its mother has become greater and with it the distance to its mother's social setting, and maybe to its siblings, aunts and uncles, etc. The problem here is the increasing age difference between the child and the previous generation. Here one may point out that fathers do not have a biological clock either and using social freezing as a means to achieve equal rights would therefore be consistent with emancipation. Yet this argument fails to note that fatherhood at a late age is hardly regarded as a moral virtue but is often seen as an egocentric decision.

All this may not suffice to prohibit social freezing. However, this reasoning makes it clear that doctors in particular must understand the urgency of informing the patient of these implications as well as of the technological options. The more couples are confronted with only the capabilities of technology without being prepared for the challenges that these technologies entail for them and their entire life, the further they will follow the escalating spiral of feasibility until they recognize far too late what they done.

Alternatives to Engineered Reproduction

Undesired childlessness has been a problem for humanity since time immemorial. A person's desire to have children is deeply seated and can cause great pain if it goes unfulfilled. History tells us of the pervasive and painful urgency of the desire to have children; it is a common theme in literature, fairy tales, and even in the Bible. There have been and still are many couples in such distress, and the fact that medicine has developed methods to help some of them is to be welcomed. To belittle this would be to trivialize the distress of couples desiring but unable to have children. To this extent, the goal cannot be to condemn the increasing use of technology per se; rather, the goal must be to ensure that technology is applied with prudence and a sense of proportion.

Alleviate Suffering

Pregnancy and birth are increasingly viewed from the perspective of simple expediency rather than leaving them in their original context of emotions that we today must relearn: feelings of excitement, respect, awe, and inspiration. Subjugating these exceptional situations in the life of a human being to the inherent imperatives of a fully rationalized, fully engineered medicine has robbed these important exceptional situations of their intrinsic meaning. Especially couples fervently desiring children or expecting a child depend on a society and a health care system to give them back these feelings so that they may again be happy people. In the face of these exceptional situations, modern medicine may well be just as speechless and helpless as our society, which is geared to efficiency and success. This speechlessness and helplessness is hidden far too quickly behind technological perfection. Where such fundamental questions of human life are involved, technology per se cannot provide the answers that many people yearn for, particularly when they are confronted with distress, abandonment, renunciation, and anxiety. Therefore, in the future it can no longer suffice to regard the areas discussed earlier simply as engineering problems but as existential crises, as situations of distress in which the people affected must not be left alone with solely technological options. On the contrary, they must be able to hope for a medical and societal system that is interested in their distress and seeks to help them in a holistic manner.

It is not "bringing about" a birth but alleviating suffering from undesired childlessness that should be the goal of humane medicine.

As long as the medical success of reproductive medicine is measured solely by the baby take-home rate, any measures that do not lead to the birth of a child appear pointless. Thus, contrary to its own promise, reproductive medicine often fails to do justice to a part of those who turn to it seeking help. With a success rate of under 20%, we can even question whether we are talking about a successful technique. Does not the feasibility quagmire ultimately cause more suffering than it promises to "master"? Many studies show that some of the couples ultimately suffer more from the repeated unsuccessful attempts than from the undesired childlessness itself.

Considering this imbalance and realizing that the context is larger than the "technological imperative" I mentioned earlier suggests, it becomes clear that the fundamental focus of humane medicine should not be the birth but the suffering of the couple. In its concentration solely on engineering expertise, medicine fails to do justice to its core task as the science of healing in the sense of the higher-order goal of alleviating a person's suffering. It neglects to turn to the person in his suffering even and indeed especially in cases where that which is feasible has reached its limits, where the suffering person needs emotional support and needs to be shown alternate perspectives. This basically applies to communicating any drastic diagnosis: the affected person's self-image is invariably plunged into a deep crisis, and it is the doctor's responsibility to perceive the suffering person in this comprehensive vulnerability and not only with respect to a functional incapacitation that may possibly be rectifiable.

Thus, reproductive medicine cannot be reduced to confronting couples having an unfulfilled desire to have children with technological options and then leaving them alone when the technology fails, possibly even with the feeling that it was not the technology that failed but they themselves. Many women experience the lack of success as a personal failure, representing a fallacious but nonetheless dramatic trans-mutation of the technological obsession into guilt (I will discuss this in Chapter 4). "I am afraid of (my body) failing." This remark is often heard and should give us pause. Comprehensive medicine in the sense described earlier would have the responsibility of not allowing technological losers to ever arise. This would not mean placing ever greater faith in the potential of technology; instead, it would mean placing what might appear to be "losing" in a broader context in those cases where technology fails.

The thought that the engineered solution might not always be the best occurs to many couples far too seldom. Medicine should make these solutions available as a matter of course, yet should always remain aware of their limits and should openly discuss the possibility of their failure with the couples. Only discussing the possibility of failure as soon and as openly as possible gives couples the chance to become comfortable with possible alternatives such as adoption, foster parenting, or even a life without children of their own. Could not humane medicine even contribute to experiencing the inability of technology to bring about a pregnancy not as a failure but as humility in the face of the ultimate immutability of the child?

> Instead of suggesting the absolute controllability and feasibility of life, we should, with respect to unborn life as well, gain back that which we may have lost the most: a fundamental attitude of humility.

The Child as a Gift and Mystery

One can only wish for a child. One cannot place an order for it. The desire to have a child must remain a wish because one can only accept a new person when one wishes. The wish expresses that it is beyond our power to determine whether it will be fulfilled. We can hope but we cannot simply order it. Even in the age of omnipresent technology, it is necessary that we do not simply calculate the person's beginning as a purely rational exercise but retain a fundamental attitude of awe. All technology notwithstanding, there is still something mysterious inherent in the beginning of a person. There is such a thing as a secret of the origin of the person and this secret demands humility of us. It also demands the understanding that the origin of a person is not to be seen as feasible but invariably as an immutable event. The philosopher Max Scheler (1874–1928) expressed it in this manner: "Humility opens the mind's eye for all the world's values. It alone, proceeding from the notion that nothing is earned and everything is a gift and a wonder, may gain everything."

This fundamental attitude of humility will also be helpful in the case of an unborn child that one subjects to prenatal diagnostics. Here, too, one will not be happy if one encounters the child solely with the fundamental attitude of doing, selecting, and disposing. The more the child is seen as something to be done, which one can decide about as desired, the more one will fail to recognize what a mystery each and every person is and what a miracle the arrival of a new human being represents.

Every unborn life touches us because it has to do with us.

A person holds his breath when a new human being comes. He is awestruck. He senses something profound. That we are deeply touched is an indication of how essential it is for our self-image as human beings to encounter the beginning of each new life with this fundamental attitude of humility.

Chapter 2
Screen, Test, Weed Out?

Never before has human freedom been held in such high esteem as it is today and never before have people had so many opportunities for choice available to them. Yet especially in dealing with prenatal diagnostics, we see that a broad range of options does not necessarily correlate with greater freedom. For is the couple expecting a baby today actually freer? This chapter examines the question of why the way we deal with unborn life today cannot make us happy. It examines the social expectation, engendered by diagnostics, of a "flawless" child and takes a look at abortion, which has been declared technological normality and whose potential for emotional and moral conflict has been relegated to private life. It advocates allowing room for suffering and presents examples of how acceptance of what is given can help us overcome crisis situations.

The Double-Edged Sword of Prenatal Diagnostics

Until a few decades ago, the coming child remained hidden. Today, we can view every detail of the unborn child's physical body. Even before it makes itself apparent with palpable movements within the mother's womb; it can be detected and diagnostically evaluated using various techniques. First there is ultrasound, which monitors its development and provides information about the shape of its body and the development of its organs. Then there are blood tests and finally what are referred to as the invasive methods (amniocentesis, chorionic villus biopsy, cordocentesis). These involve direct intervention into the uterus to remove cells from the unborn child, which are then subjected to laboratory tests for certain genetic anomalies or diseases.

There are two sides to these increasing possibilities for learning something about the child. Prenatal diagnostic modalities undoubtedly represent a blessing where they contribute to early detection of disease in the mother or child and thus allow early onset of treatment. Such is the case in rhesus incompatibility between the mother and child or insufficient nutrient supply to the fetus from the placenta. However, the options for early treatment apply to only a fraction of the cases. The great majority of disorders and disabilities detected by prenatal diagnostics are not treatable. Once a pregnancy occurs, couples are faced with the nearly unbearable ethical conflict of continuing the pregnancy under the unfavorable condition of a diagnosed anomaly or "terminating" it, which means nothing other than deciding whether the child will live or die. In addition to this, the opportunity to detect an untreatable disease or disability in an unborn child burdens the parents with a certain societal expectation, namely that of a "healthy" child, whereas the acceptance of a "disabled" child decreases correspondingly. Given these examination modalities, the parents can simply no longer afford to accept the child as it is. They are expected, more or less tacitly, to screen the child where techniques are available for this purpose. Couples today are thus ultimately expected to ensure that they bring "flawless" children into the world. If they do not do so, they have done something wrong and are regarded as negligent and irresponsible.

A Patient's Story

I would like to introduce the problems of prenatal diagnostics by recounting a patient's story in which I became involved as a disinterested party and which has given me pause.

A 29-year-old woman had developed what is known as a gestosis, a pathological disorder of pregnancy during her first pregnancy. This disorder was so severe that the patient's life was threatened. However, adequate medical care successfully brought it under control. The disorder nonetheless resulted in a premature birth. In the 24th week of pregnancy she delivered a child weighing less than 500 grams. Thanks to medical technology the child was able to survive all complications and developed well. Today it is 6 years old. Three years ago, the patient became pregnant a second time. She took prophylactic medications to prevent a second gestosis. However, an ultrasound examination in the 18th week of pregnancy revealed that the unborn child was significantly undernourished and had developed an extreme growth impairment, which can be a typical picture for such a pregnancy disorder. The examining gynecologist emphasized that the child most probably would not survive and advised the patient to terminate the pregnancy as waiting for the fetus to die in the uterus would be too great a burden for the pregnant woman. The patient categorically refused an abortion and went to the university medical center. Here, they confirmed the very serious prognosis for the child but left the question unanswered as to whether an abortion would be the proper decision in this situation. Strengthened in her conviction, the patient resolved to continue the pre-gnancy, albeit under the strict supervision of a doctor.

The pregnancy initially progressed without any complications under medical therapy. However, a cesarean section had to be performed in the 22nd week of pregnancy due to the poor nourishment of the fetus. This was the only way to prevent the death of the infant in the uterus.

The child came into world weighing 430 grams; it required artificial respiration and had to be placed in an incubator. The chance of survival was very slight, although there was hope that the child might be saved, seeing as the firstborn child had been able to recover completely from a minimally higher weight 3 years previously. The situation initially appeared stable but the findings worsened dramatically on the third day. The decision was finally made to refrain from additional measures and the child was allowed to die peacefully.

The parents parted from their child with great pain. Even today, years later, they have not yet overcome this loss. They have decided against a third pregnancy. In spite of this, the parents experienced the 3 days that they were able to spend with their son.

This patient's story clearly reveals the double-edged nature of prenatal diagnostics. The opportunity for such diagnostics was certainly of great value for this young woman. Without it the child would have been in a significantly more threatening situation and probably would have died in the uterus. In this way, it was also possible for her to acquire a realistic picture of the complications to be expected. But prenatal diagnostics also has its drawbacks. Its very existence alone forced a decision on the parents that never would have had to have been made without such an examination: the decision as to whether this child should continue to live or whether action should be taken to end its life beforehand. The young woman categorically rejected the doctor's recommendation to have an abortion because she saw life as a gift and could not conceive of taking action to end it herself. However, her story makes it clear how easily people in this situation can be confronted with the dilemma of an abortion if the prenatal examination produces an accumulation of negative findings.

What would be a foregone conclusion without prenatal diagnostics, namely that a child lives as long as it is able to live, becomes a personal choice with the availability of diagnostics.

The end of this patient's story shows what a difference it makes whether one kills a child oneself or whether one allows it to die. This couple decided categorically to watch and wait and to leave it to nature, fate, or God to determine whether or not the child may continue to live. The abortion recommended by the doctor would have caused at least this mother enormous feelings of guilt while denying her the experience of seeing her own child even if only for a few days. Every story stands for itself. It cannot be generalized, yet it reveals a lot.

First I would like to note that it is indeed advisable and necessary to place the unborn child under the supervision of a doctor. The purpose of prenatal diagnostics is not primarily to raise the question of abortion. On the contrary, the actual and original purpose lay, and lies, in the early detection of developmental disorders so as to facilitate early treatment of the child where possible. Properly applied, these examinations also serve to allay the fears and worries of the pregnant woman and to give her certainty while preparing her for the further course of pregnancy.

Offering prenatal diagnostics is thus a part of the doctor's obligation to exercise due diligence. Nonetheless, it has its drawbacks. These do not arise from prenatal diagnostics as such but ultimately result from its use. The more routine screening the unborn child becomes and the more detailed the information obtained about the child becomes, the more we achieve the opposite of what good prenatal diagnostics should do. Because when applied without reflection according to a standardized scheme, prenatal diagnostics does not lead to the desired certainty but often unsettles the pregnant woman. This can become a severe burden, and often even the slightest diagnostic uncertainty leads to precautionary termination of the pregnancy. Rather than taking a risk, having an abortion still seems to be the safest way to prevent a child with disabilities.

Expecting, but No Longer with Anticipation

Although intrinsically beneficial, prenatal diagnostics reveals its downside where pregnancy, once viewed positively, becomes a problematic condition. This begins with the classification of a pregnancy as a "high-risk pregnancy," which is the point of entry and justification for prenatal diagnostics.

So-called high-risk patients include pregnant women who:
- *are older than 35 years;*
- *already have one child with a chromosome abnormality;*
- *have a familial predisposition for disorders detectable by prenatal diagnostics;*
- *have shown abnormal findings at the routine ultrasound examination.*

The unborn child as a symbol of hope for a new light, for a person who could change the world: this view is effectively blocked in today's world of prenatal monitoring. What the indiscriminate application of prenatal diagnostics achieves is the loss of an unbiased approach to pregnancy. This often means that in our minds we divide it into two phases. Initially we have a conditional pregnancy; it only becomes an acceptable pregnancy once prenatal diagnostics has revealed normal findings. Paradoxically, this downgrading of pregnancy from what was once a state of anticipation is associated with a question that is still largely tabooed: when actually confronted with the diagnosis of disease or disability, how do parents cope with the challenge of having to decide whether their child will live or die?

This is confirmed by a project sponsored by the EU since 2005 to examine the effects of genetic and prenatal diagnostics on pregnant women and their partners. The study shows how traumatizing the decision conflict is for the people involved.[11] Another study primarily based on reports of personal experience also came to the conclusion that as long as it confirms the hope of having a normal child, prenatal diagnostics as a routine option is the talk of the town. However, findings that might actually deviate from the norm as well as possible consequences are tabooed by both the environment in general and the doctors involved.[12] One young woman describes it in these words: "You think the examination is routine but then suddenly the earth stops turning."[13] She confirms the findings of a representative study of prenatal diagnostics commissioned by the German Federal Office of Health Education (BZgA) in 2004. That study dramatically illustrated that pregnant women, despite their increasing use of these examinations, basically do not know what consequences the examinations might entail.

Having personally experienced the ethical dilemma of prenatal diagnostics, film producer and television editor Monika Hey has written an impressive book on the subject whose German title translates as *My Glass Belly: How Prenatal Diagnostics Changes Our*

Relationship to Life. She has compiled a list of questions about the individual examination methods which represents the minimum that the pregnant woman should be clear about prior to the respective examination:

- What does the diagnostics involve?
- When is it used?
- What do I learn?
- What is there to consider? (What consequences are associated with this knowledge? What possibly unjustified anxieties?)[14]

From this alone, it becomes clear what great responsibility the physician must bear when performing prenatal diagnostics. Because even the way in which the physician communicates the findings will decisively influence the pregnant woman's decision whether to have an abortion or to give birth to the child.

In my opinion, the ethical responsibility of modern medicine consists in undertaking to avoid fully sacrificing the pregnant woman's lightheartedness and impartiality and in avoiding a pathological mindset with respect to pregnancy in the sense of representing it as a disease. The more findings are collected, the more prenatal life is threatened. For, with every finding, one is asked the question: Do you want the child anyway? Anyway! This "anyway" is dangerous because it expresses the idea that one must justify deciding in favor of life and not against it. That is the crux of the matter.

What we have here is a reversal of the meaning of responsible parenthood. Responsible parenthood increasingly means that one monitors sufficiently and only says yes to life when the examination findings have been negative. When abnormal findings occur, then saying yes to life essentially requires justification. That is what this "anyway" means. Saying yes to life means increasingly running the risk that others will not find it plausible given the knowledge of a disease, of a disability, or of a simple deviation from the norm. Saying yes to life is no longer the most self-evident and humane thing to do but is increasingly becoming a daring decision. Wolfram Henn, professor of human genetics at the University of Saarland, has expressed this in similar terms:

> "We are increasingly succumbing—the more so, the more options there are—to what I would almost call a delusion of feasibility, that we increasingly believe that we can guarantee healthy children with medicine. That is not true at all. And we must work against and advise against this attitude of entitlement. And in particular we must continue to give parents who say, 'I would like to remain in good hope,' to phrase it biblically, that very chance. We must defend the right to say no with tooth and nail."[15]

Is the Handicapped Child an Avoidable Risk?

Looking at current developments, we can readily see how important this reasoning is. The Praena test is a blood test developed by the LifeCodexx AG company in Konstanz, Germany, that has been available since August 2012. Starting with the 10th week of pregnancy, this test can be used without risk to the mother or child to determine whether the unborn child has trisomy 21.

Trisomy 21 or Down's syndrome is one of the most commonly occurring chromosome anomalies in newborns. The 21st chromosome or parts of it are present in triplicate. People with this developmental anomaly thus have 47 chromosomes in each cell of their body instead of the usual 46. Unlike many other chromosome anomalies that lead to early miscarriages (which often go unnoticed), trisomy 21 does not usually impair the development of the embryo. Down's syndrome is a genetic deviation from the normal condition and not a disease. Generally trisomy 21 is associated with conspicuous physical characteristics and a slight to moderate limitation of cognitive capabilities. About 50,000 people live with Down's syndrome in Germany.

The Blood Test for Trisomy 21

In contrast to the conventional invasive methods (chorionic villus biopsy, amniocentesis) that always entail the risk inherent in any intervention, this noninvasive method represents progress. Disregarding the ethical reservations, it simply combines two commonly practiced procedures: the first trimester screening that almost every pregnant woman undergoes (consisting of an ultrasound examination and a blood test measuring proteins) and the amniotic fluid analysis previously reserved for high-risk patients (which it does without risk).

At first glance, one could think that the blood test should clearly be viewed positively. Replacing amniocentesis, which is associated with a mortality rate for the child of up to 1%, is indisputably a high moral goal. How can one criticize a method that can spare the lives of 300 children per year when we proceed from the 30,000 amniocentesis procedures that are currently performed annually? And yet we must also consider the larger context in order to come to a more nuanced understanding of the test. That means that we must not ignore the laudable characteristics of the Praena test while at the same time refraining from dismissing the test as simply harmless. Regarding it as harmless seems obvious because the advantages are so evident and the problems the test entails are only very subtle.

As paradoxical as it may sound, the Praena test becomes dangerous precisely because it is so simple and easily performed. Because it is associated with a promise. It promises safety and certainty as long as we can proceed from negative findings. Even this is misleading because the test does not tell us that the child is healthy. It only excludes a certain form of disability. Positive findings, on the other hand, often plunge the pregnant woman unprepared into a situation in which she suddenly has to answer a question of life and death. The danger is that the pregnant woman only becomes aware of the full significance of this seemingly harmless blood test when she can no longer ignore the results.

But is that not a situation that we have with every prenatal diagnostic test, and with amniocentesis as well? It is completely correct that the decision situations into which the pregnant women are thrust are the same in both cases. The particular difference lies in the fact that am-niocentesis, precisely because it is dangerous, sets in motion a different reflection process from the outset than does the blood test. Women tend to approach the decision to undergo amniocentesis cautiously, circumspectly, and critically. And it is good that they do. One automatically contemplates the possible consequences of this in-tervention because it is impossible to avoid considering them when making the decision. However, the Praena test suggests that such difficult reflection in advance is no longer required at all as this is only a harmless blood test. Should this test gradually establish itself as a "filtering method" it will become dangerous. The danger is not inherent in the test itself but in the counseling that may not be given due consideration where the test is applied automatically. That at least is the first danger.

The second danger posed by the Praena test is also related to the tendency to apply the test on a broad scale, yet this danger is more subtle. Were the test to become a standard component of prenatal diagnostics, it would have enormous effects, not only on the women in question but also with respect to society, effects that the health care system must be prepared to contemplate. Because it will depend on doctors whether the Praena test will be used only in individual cases in which there is an existing risk profile or whether it will gradually become normal practice in every pregnancy. First, we could say that the company's marketing strategy has been successful. The test was introduced very cautiously and that has also ensured its broad acceptance. Cautiously, because it is initially intended only for pregnant women with an increased individual risk, because it should be applied only after the 12th week of pregnancy, and also because it is relatively expensive and the statutory health insurance funds do not assume these costs. However, these restrictions presumably cannot be maintained in the long term. Because why should one neglect the far larger group of "low-risk pregnancies," especially in light of economic interests?

Its simplicity and easy application could turn the test into a routine procedure in the long term and encourage its unrestricted use. "The safer diagnostic procedures become, the greater is the probability that they will be routinely used,"[16] as Markus Dederich, rehabilitation specialist and educator for the disabled in Cologne, has so succinctly put it. The danger exists that the Praena test could soon become established as a screening method, that is to say a systematic test procedure for filtering. And that would mean that the test would be implicitly understood as an instrument that "prevents" the birth of children with Down's syndrome to the greatest extent possible. Down's syndrome, in its clinical picture rather undramatic for the person affected compared with other disabilities, would in this way become the first form of disability to disappear from society by means of systematic detection and abortion, as Wolfram Henn has critically remarked. Here physicians bear a great responsibility because it is ultimately up to them whether this test will signify an increase in opportunities or an increase in problems.

Searching for Nonconforming Life?

The physician's genuine decision lives from, and its good is precisely measured by, the fact that it attempts to give an answer to the affected pregnant woman relative to her respective unique situation. The core task of obstetrics and gynecology is to attend to pregnant women, to help them, and to stand by them with good advice. The concept of medicine as the healing science shows that for the physician as a representative of a social profession, the focus of every action must invariably be on the entire human being. Healing science does not mean providing a service, it means interpersonal care. The decision to perform amniocentesis is in the best case the result of many consultations and reflections which primarily revolve around the question of how best to help the woman and the unborn child. This help can involve still being able to do something for the child when it is found to have a disorder or providing help for the pregnant woman as well and especially for her so that she can prepare for the child and can reflect on her own resilience.

Were we now to allow the blood test for trisomy 21 to become a routine examination, then this would no longer be a singular decision relating to a unique situation. Instead, it would be a standard procedure that by virtue of its standardization conveys a message. And this is: it is good and laudable to undergo this test not only in individual situations but also as a matter of course. Yet if it is good to perform this test as a matter of course, then we will be saying nothing else than that it is good and right to protect oneself against a child with trisomy 21. The routine use of the Praena test is associated with the implicit tendency to regard life with Down's syndrome as a fundamentally avoidable "evil." This implicit message is as concealed as it is dangerous. For it suggests that medicine's task is no longer primarily about helping people in distress but simply about a search for ostensibly nonconforming life.

But why should medicine search for "nonconforming" life? After all, trisomy 21 is not a disorder that can be treated. If the blood test for trisomy 21 is determined to be medically indicated solely because trisomy 21 represents a genetic disability, then this is nothing other than a subtle form of eugenics. It means that the physician basically no longer regards the unborn child in its intrinsic individuality but as a genetic finding. That in turn means that if the Praena test were to become routine, medicine itself would have expressed the belief that life with Down's syndrome is an evil that reason dictates must be prevented. The implicit message that it is natural to search for this chromosome anomaly is fateful because one thereby does nothing less than pass a negative judgment on this life, and does that as a physician!

Here one could legitimately object that it is not medicine that demands this test but society, which ultimately demands from medicine that it ensure that only healthy children come into the world. Thus, it is more the social expectation than medicine itself that represents the fundamental problem. Here we should first consider that there is a connection between social expectation and the range of medical options. It is medicine's diagnostic options and especially the tendency to play down these options that give rise to such expectations in the first place. For precisely this reason, it is part of the physician's responsibility to consider in advance what social effects certain medical interventions and diagnostic procedures will entail so as to prevent the worst by applying these options circumspectly.

All of this reasoning is intended to illustrate the social context in which medicine operates. We live in an age in which the social expectation placed on pregnant women is so powerful that the medical profession would make it too easy for itself by regarding itself as merely a service provider and simply fulfilling people's desire to have children. On the contrary, today more than ever medicine must remain a place of help and care. The physician is ultimately someone who does not act on the basis of desires to have children, but according to principles. And the core principle must be that medicine can only act for the good of the pregnant woman and the child. Medicine can ultimately achieve this only by accepting the pregnant woman in her confusion and helplessness and by attempting to be not merely a service provider but a wise counselor.

The Praena test requires the physician to give wise advice. And he can only give such advice after interacting with the pregnant woman and out of deep respect for her freedom. Yet this freedom of the pregnant woman must first be built, it cannot simply be called upon. The physician's task is to help the future mother make a carefully considered decision which in the best case will have a lifelong effect. The physician must refrain from patronizing, for it would be wrong to understand care as acting solely on behalf of the child and simply advising the woman not to undergo a test. Nor would it be wise advice for the physician to suggest that the Praena test is obviously indicated simply because the physician regards it as rational or reasonable.

On the contrary, the consultation must remain open-ended, which does not mean that one remains indifferent. A good physician must not remain indifferent but must see the pregnant woman's distress as a mission requiring the physician's personal dedication in order to find a good solution together with the pregnant woman or the future parents. Thus, the physician's task includes first clarifying what it really means to have a child with Down's syndrome. The physician should advise the pregnant woman to obtain a realistic and comprehensive picture of life with this disability, for example, by establishing contact with affected families or self-help groups. This is because most women who abort such a child have only rudimentary experiences with these children. They act in response to an internalized social expectation. In other words, obstetrics and gynecology would be betraying pregnant women to suggest there is a simple answer to their distress because society expects only one answer from them. On the contrary, medicine must provide a compassionate medical consultation to strengthen the women's resolve so that they can make a decision that corresponds to their own concept of life.

Preimplantation Genetic Diagnostics: Is a Child a Product under Warranty?

The increasing technological diagnostic options do not mean simply an increase in freedom of choice; they can also represent a narrowing of choices by prematurely blocking alternate paths. This is apparent in the development of prenatal diagnostics but even more strikingly in the preimplantation genetic diagnostics (PGD) so heatedly discussed in the media, that is, in the type of diagnostics applied prior to the actual pregnancy. PGD involves genetic testing of artificially fertilized eggs so that only embryos that do not show a genetic disposition for severe disorders are transferred to the uterus. PGD also provides the opportunity to pick out one of many embryos. It implies a choice; we could also refer to a selection. This represents a selection decision in which a person decides which embryo may live and which may not.

The debate in Germany about PGD began with this patient history:

> *A married couple came to a gynecologist with the following previous history: 5 years previously, the couple had been confronted with the birth of a child with severe cystic fibrosis, an incurable metabolic disease. The child died shortly after birth. Genetic testing revealed that both parents were carriers of a mutation in the respective gene. A new pregnancy would entail a 25% risk of recurrence. A second pregnancy occurred. The couple wanted to avoid a second death right after birth and decided to undergo prenatal diagnostics with amniocentesis. The findings were positive, and the couple decided to terminate the pregnancy. A third pregnancy occurred. Again amniocentesis was performed, again the findings were positive, and again the pregnancy was terminated. The couple consulted a gynecologist and asked whether they could be helped by PGD.*

The case in Lübeck, Germany, described above graphically illustrates how medicine with the expansion of its genetic testing options not only "solves" existing problems but also creates new problems and poses new questions. May a genetic test be performed on an embryo as a kind of preliminary prenatal diagnostics? In other words, as long as we can examine everything in the mother's uterus and reject and abort life after prenatal diagnostics, how can we simultaneously raise objections to PGD?

The fundamental problem of PGD is that an embryo is in fact conceived but is only kept alive under the condition that it is not the carrier of a certain genetic defect. Thus, the embryo is conceived on probation and its acceptance is made conditional not on its existence but on a genetic quality test. The embryo can only live if it passes the test. The problematic aspect of this act arises not only from that fact that the right to life of the embryo is called into question, but also from the fact that human life in this case is conceived on probation and is not unconditionally accepted with respect to its genetic makeup. Prenatal genetic diagnostics itself has already seen the widespread acceptance of an attitude toward unborn life that no longer regards the genetic state of unborn life as given, but as controllable and as an object to be controlled by human decisions. The expanding diagnostic options have increasingly made the unborn child subject to the logic of "quality control." As we have seen, the child must pass tests increasingly often before a definitive decision is made in its favor and thus in favor of its life. PGD can in fact be understood as the continuation of this thinking, albeit in a totally new dimension because the selection of the "desirable" embryos is factored in from the outset and does not remain limited to extreme cases.

As such thinking progresses, it changes our attitude toward the unborn children and thus our attitude to ourselves as well. Children are increasingly understood as products that we order, evaluate according to quality criteria, and send back if we do not like them. What is lost is the feeling of gratitude for the hidden child that has come into being. This feeling is being supplanted by fear, the fear of insufficient control. The child thus becomes the result of our own evaluation criteria, a product that we only accept if it meets the specified requirements and quality standards. Nothing different applies to PGD. Here the embryos are only conceived on probation and only the quality test in the form of the genetic examination decides whether we will accept the product or reject it for poor quality.

At first glance, this appears to be an increase in freedom, being able to choose instead of having to accept an unchosen fate. Yet, when we look more closely, it becomes apparent that the increased freedom of choice also involves a loss of freedom; being able to choose increasingly means having to choose. Each instance of having to choose also leads to an increase in fallibility and potential tragedy. Widespread acceptance of PGD indeed does not lead to everyone being able to choose freely whether or not they want this diagnostic testing. On the contrary, it gives rise to social pressure to actually avail oneself of these examination options. There is another aspect to be considered as well: the possible decisions thrust an enormous responsibility on the individual, the responsibility for the fact that this unwanted child is rejected, that now that child exists and not another. Moreover, technological achievements are always praised and marketed as new freedoms, yet people fail to see that these are freedoms that have been gained at someone else's expense. A genuine freedom can only be one gained with the other person and not at his expense.

Ultimately, even the freedom of those suffers who have survived the selection in the test tube or the mother's womb. Because those embryos selected for survival will later live with the knowledge that they were conceived but initially not accepted. Unfavorable genetic findings would have meant their death. The embryo that was not rejected will later know that he lives not because he is unique but because he passed a test. The notion that his parents would not have accepted a life with him as a handicapped child would be a burden because he could think that there may come a time when he is no longer good enough for his parents, for example, if he should become sick. This reveals what would be the price of giving up an unconditional acceptance of life. It reveals how much a human being needs to live in the knowledge that his life is something given and not something chosen.

As long as a practice is accepted in which the life in the mother's womb is conditional on the decision of the future parents, it appears implausible and counterintuitive that we will now erect high barriers in dealing with embryos conceived in vitro. The following cynical remark has made the rounds among gynecologists: "The embryo is protected in the test tube until it can be aborted in the uterus." There is some truth to this sentence when one observes only the practice. Thus, there are only two options. The first is to permit PID under the law in light of current practice. Then we would have to establish why the embryo may be used as an object, why it should receive its right to live only by virtue of its parents' good will, and why total disposition over prenatal life should be unproblematic. The second is to establish political precedents clearly indicating that neither the routine selection of persons in mother's uterus nor the freedom of disposition over prenatal life in the form of a probationary pregnancy is in keeping with the law.

> On July 7, 2011, the German Bundestag voted by a clear majority to declare PID prohibited in principle but permissible in exceptional cases. These exceptional cases are deemed to exist when a high probability of a severe hereditary disease is present or the danger exists that the pregnancy will end in a miscarriage or stillbirth. Requirements for PGD include a prior consultation and the approval of the Ethics Commission.

The problem of PGD as I see it is that embryos are conceived on probation and subjected to a quality test before we decide in their favor. In so doing, we indicate that we do not accept life unconditionally but only that life which fulfills certain criteria we have chosen. From an ethical standpoint, this raises the question of whether prenatal diagnostics departed from the unconditional acceptance of every life even before PGD. Even if it could be said that the practice of prenatal diagnostics already embodies just such thinking, then we would have to consider whether we could consider such a practice good. In any case, a tendency to increasingly subject unborn life to systematic control is evident. And all the technological "achievements" mentioned are moving in precisely this direction. They are initially praised as an increase in freedom but they implicitly lead to an ever more powerful social expectation to actually avail oneself of these examination options.

It is no longer sufficient to simply be happy to have a child because one must not only have a child, any child, but invariably a successful child, a child sufficiently well prepared to hold its own in a competitive society. The responsibility for doing so is implicitly thrust on the parents. Yet, in fact, they thrust it upon themselves if they are of the opinion that they themselves can determine whether or not the child will be happy. And it can only be happy if it wins the "battle" against the others. In our age, parents put themselves under enormous pressure and naturally pass this on to their children. The dramatic thing about this is that this pressure is exerted long before birth.

Apparently, it is no longer sufficient to find ways to aid the child years after its birth. The responsibility for aiding the child begins with the existence of the child in the mother's womb or even in the test tube. We mold the child into a winner even before its birth as if it were the most natural thing in the world. Everything that could stand in the way of becoming a winner is swept aside even at the expense of the life of the unborn person itself. One gynecologist expresses it in these terms:

"Do we not actually now have an alliance for selection, never referred to as such since the word has overly negative connotations, but tolerated by society and implemented by the physicians?"[17]

That may sound somewhat overstated but I am convinced that we have already internalized this creed in many areas without realizing it. Maybe we really do not want to admit this because it would be uncomfortable to do so. Yet, it is important to think about this because our age offers so many freedoms and options insofar as we put them to use in a prudent and truly genuine manner.

The Gray Area between Demand and Taboo: Abortion

When we talk about the ethical limits of prenatal diagnostics and PID, we cannot avoid taking a closer look at abortion. The liberation of abortion is in no small measure the background against which a practice of prenatal diagnostics such as that we described has been able to develop. The expansion of prenatal diagnostics has ultimately been driven by the realization that we can always have an abortion. Without abortion as a socially acceptable method, prenatal diagnostics with all its unsettling consequences would certainly never have experienced this expansion.

In the 1970s, it was regarded as a milestone of humane policy that abortion was decriminalized and could even be performed legally when the woman's health was at risk. Decades later we sense that legal liberalization has hardly solved all the severe problems of abortion. The feeling in the 1970s was it was the woman's right to decide for herself whether or not to have an abortion. At that time we could hardly have predicted that this legal empowerment would not actually give every woman the freedom to decide herself. Monika Hey puts it in a nutshell when she emphasizes, "As pregnant women we face a well-organized medical system which we know far too little about. Pregnancy is the worst time to think about the issues of pre-natal diagnostics. Women must be better informed in advance so as to be able to defend themselves against what prenatal diagnostics will confront them with. They should be able to do what they want and not what they are supposed to want."[18]

Today abortion is regarded as possible and that also means that a woman does not have to have any unwanted children. And if she has them anyway, then it is her own fault so to speak because she could "very easily" have decided to have an abortion. This applies especially to our behavior toward children with disabilities. Whoever has a handicapped child today will be asked why the woman did not have an abortion, especially since it would have been so easy. This also applies to the number of children, the time of birth, and so on. Today it is a person's own fault for having many children or having them at the "wrong" time because it would have been easy to abort them. The "project-specific child," as sociologist Luc Boltanski calls it, is denied access to life when the "parent project" demands it in the setting of a "project-based society."[19]

The option of abortion in our age is understood to mean that we can determine the time of birth, the number, and the health of the chil-dren ourselves. In addition to this, the liberalization of abortion has led to a situation in which the pregnant woman's social setting, but primarily her partner, has enormous influence over her. Thirty-nine percent of the women interviewed in one study responded that the decision to have an abortion was made primarily in the face of press-ure from their environment.[20] Many women hardly have a chance to resist their partner's pressure in their condition and given their pre-carious social situation. Often they give in and almost as often their relationships fail or at least cool down.

People fought hard to allow abortion. Yet the freedom to abort has put the pregnant woman at the mercy of the external expectation to prefer abortion to having a child that her partner or her social setting in general does not want at the moment. Despite all the euphoria about the liberalization of abortion, the pregnant women and future mothers themselves have been radically abandoned with no thought given to their emotional state, as has now, years later, been borne out by numerous reports of personal experience and scientific studies, especially by women.

The Emotional Consequences of Abortion Are Taboo

Many studies show that many women who have had an abortion later have to struggle with emotional problems. They grieve for their children who were killed and struggle with their fate. Psychologist Maria Simon described the emotional late sequelae of abortion as follows: "feelings of remorse and guilt, self-recrimination, mood swings and depression, tears for no reason, anxiety, and nightmares."[21] Many relationships fail because of this, and many women later blame it on their physicians. They do this partly in an attempt to suppress their own responsibility but also partly because they rightfully feel betrayed by them. They struggle with the fact that the physician did not tell them about the late sequelae of abortion and they struggle especially with the fact that they gave in too quickly to the recommendation to have an abortion. One affected woman described it like this, "The doctors decided over my head. They frightened me into thinking the child could be impaired. If I were in the same situation again, I would give birth even if my child were impaired. It is my flesh and blood. I would love it."[22] Another woman reported, "The doctor told me [...] the embryo might be impaired. I don't know if that was true. For fear of the child's disability that was being suggested to me I had the pregnancy terminated. I would have loved to have had the child."[23]

It must give us pause that, as studies show, 42% of the women interviewed after having an abortion later question their decision and are often plagued by the futile wish to undo the abortion.[24] Other studies show a similarly high percentage of later depression, especially in women who aborted at a young age.[25] Certainly, one should always be very cautious in interpreting such figures and in constructing causal relationships. It must also be remembered that the severity of the emotional sequelae always depends as well on what social support the women receive, how they are cared for, and how they are prepared for the abortion. Nonetheless, these findings make it clear that, while the degree may vary, it is not at all true that abortion has no lasting effect on women's emotional sensitivity. The fact that this topic has still been largely ignored is due in no small measure to the fact that many affected women do not dare to speak about it openly. That in turn is because abortion, although expected, is simultaneously tabooed. It is regarded as an entirely personal decision that the woman alone bears responsibility for. Accordingly, other people such as family members, friends, or coworkers are less willing to listen to complaints about the negative effects of the abortion. Society delegates responsibility for the abortion and its sequelae to the individual woman, who must come to terms with her struggles and feelings of guilt by herself. That is the downside of liberalization.

> The notion that a woman has complete freedom to decide as she pleases obscures the fact that unsolved ethical and social problems associated with modern technologies are being thrust on the pregnant woman.

It is also becoming increasingly obvious that a woman's decision to have an abortion is often not at all as clear as many people believe. Numerous studies suggest that many pregnant women are initially confused and in distress. They seek people who will help them and

55

support them. Unfortunately, these women encounter a health care system that is driven far too rarely by the motivation to help but all too often recommends abortion as the best solution. Many women report how quickly their doctors in particular broach the topic of abortion and how doctors are often not wise advisors but agitators.[26]

This is very disconcerting and only comprehensible when we realize that in today's medicine there is a tendency to view every deviation from the norm as a catastrophe and that the occupational socialization that physicians undergo trains them to fear this deviation and combat it with every available means. They see normal findings but fail to see the human being behind them. Gynecologists in particular also fear that the woman they are to advise today could bring legal action against them tomorrow. Far too often there have been court cases in which physicians have been sued for damages because the women accuse them of not having sufficiently informed them about the severity of the forthcoming disability or about further diagnostic options. These litigating women, according to their argumentation, would otherwise have had an abortion. There is something barbaric about the normality of abortion, but it can be used as a weapon against the physician. And many argue in this manner: because the physician did not offer them all possible diagnostic methods, they now have a child they would rather have killed. Many physicians must now pay damages not because children have been injured or killed as a result of their actions but because the physicians' culpable behavior has spared the lives of certain children whose parents say they would definitely have killed. Failure to inform the patient is indeed malpractice.

But in this setting many gynecologists are afraid of their patients because such a legal system effectively puts them at their mercy. The consequence is that many physicians, although luckily not all, disregard the best interests of both the pregnant woman and the unborn children by "aggravating" them. That means that they present the nonconforming or unclear findings as more dramatic than they actually are so that they cannot be sued later. And they often recommend an abortion in the presence of even the smallest uncertainty because the dead child is the best guarantee of avoiding charges. A physician will not be prosecuted if he convinces a woman to kill the possibly nonconforming child she is carrying but he will be severely punished if he negligently forgets certain information when obtaining the pregnant woman's informed consent. Modern medicine now finds itself in this situation of reassessing the value of a human life. Thus, it is no surprise that many women do not perceive their doctors as wise counselors but as strategists guided by interests at the expense of unborn life and at the expense of the emotional balance of many women who must struggle with their decision for many years after their abortion.

Allowing Room for Suffering

We live in a world that allows more individual freedoms than ever before. No conventions, no strict moral laws, and no binding religious tenets seem to apply any more. Modern man appears to be able to do what he wants. And the political system even supports him in this. Yet at the same time man is also the prisoner of very subtle social demands on himself. It is no longer explicitly stated that "society" today expects more from the individual than ever before, namely nothing less than his success. And this is measured according to the criteria of a competitive society that knows almost exclusively economic values: performance and production capability, efficiency, usefulness, and functionality. The individual must first demonstrate that he is functional and useful in order to be accepted as a valuable person. He is not only condemned to be himself or make something of himself, as the French existentialist Jean-Paul Sartre (1905–1980) put it, he is also condemned to be a winner, a winner in the competition for the most successful life (see also Chapter 3, p. 62).

Children with disabilities contradict this success postulate. And whoever does not succeed in "preventing" them becomes one of the losers. Yet it seems to me that the real losers are those people who do not resist this success postulate and cannot withstand the pressure to conform. These are the weak people who go against their heart and conform because they think they have no other choice. Seeking superficially to escape the realm of suffering by attempting to undo what is done, they are only drawn into it from behind all the more emphatically (as the respective studies show).

One example of the strength with which critical situations can be overcome if one only accepts them and literally carries them to term is found in the documentary film whose German title translates as *My Little Child* by midwife and film producer Katja Baumgarten. The film records her pregnancy with a severely disabled child until his birth and death (www.meinkleineskind.de). After her unborn son was found to have a complex deformity syndrome and was expected to die during pregnancy or shortly after birth, she decided against an abortion and in favor of carrying the child to term. She gave birth to the child in the circle of her closest friends and family where it was able to die peacefully in her arms a few hours later. In an interview Katja Baumgarten spoke of the "exceptional" character of this time: "As short as it was, this was a very great time for us. […] The time of the pregnancy, where I knew he would live a short time, I still tried to show him the most beautiful things in life. And then these three and a half hours, too, that was a very special time. […] Everyone greeted him. […] Even when he died, everyone was there. That was really a very deep and beautiful experience."[27] Monika Hey also writes about the consolation that can lie in being able to suffer. In her book, she quotes an unnamed human geneticist as saying:

> "I think that is ultimately more consoling to hold a child in your arms after birth and accompany it as it dies than to forcibly prevent it from living and dying by removing it prematurely. There are things that you cannot do but can only let happen and, actively, suffer through. But that also means allowing room for the happening and the suffering, in other words accepting what comes and what is not in your hands. And then in this suffering there are also consoling moments in which to do something. To accept what is grave and inevitable, to make room for sorrow, to somehow live it well, to somehow manage it in mutual sympathy and support."[28]

Taking a Stand

What I have termed the "success postulate" is unobtrusively accompanied by an increasingly pervasive mindset which, now that abortion has become technological normality, simply relegates its potential for emotional and moral conflict to private life. Yet when the life of a third party is at stake, we can no longer speak of a matter of private life because then it becomes a social and societal matter. Abortion poses the question of how we as a society want to deal with the life that cannot defend itself. It poses the question of how we can manage to apply the principle of compassion as a fundamental principle of all action to best advantage. And it poses the question of whether compassion should not be particularly evident in our dealings with the weakest members of society.

The sensitivity to the needs of people with disabilities is far greater today than 30 years ago. That is cause for hope. Something has changed in our world with respect to social issues. The greatest obstacle for unborn life is not the mother who would "much rather" kill her child. That does not correspond to reality. On the contrary, the greatest obstacle is the social expectation, internalized by many pregnant women, of never giving birth to a baby with disabilities. That is the real problem in our society. The current social climate is double-edged. On the one hand, it explicitly demands greater inclusion of people with disabilities. On the other hand, it implicitly promotes an atmosphere in which pregnant women are increasingly hesitant to say yes to their child if a disability appears to be diagnosable. This represents nothing other than exclusion prior to birth.

Now one might conclude that acceptance of disabled persons is only a facade to conceal our modern performance society's fundamentally eugenic attitude. Yet that does not correspond to reality. The signals of so many people who have devoted their entire lives to serving the good of people with disabilities are simply far too genuine and promising. Presumably, there are numerous women who neither belong to one sharply defined side or the other but are simply uncertain, simply do exactly know what they should do, and who hesitate, struggle, doubt, and occasionally despair.

These women deserve broad support in society. Many couples frantically seek signals within society, signs from its midst telling them that society declares its solidarity with them in their time of distress. These women and families need financial aid when they bring a child with a disability into the world so that they know they can live under good conditions even with a disabled child. But above all they need moral support. They need a climate in which they in particular receive the highest moral recognition and which honors the humaneness behind the attitude of saying yes to life. Many couples would commit to having a child with a disability if they know that nobody would come tomorrow and accuse them of ostensibly irresponsible behavior.

What the public thinks of couples that consciously decide in favor of a disabled child—because they see it as a gift and not a "product"—depends in no small measure on the political signals. If the political system behaves as if selecting children were progressive, then it will promote further rejection of unborn life. If, however, it goes beyond mere lip service to encourage women and couples, then it will enable couples to make a decision that they can stand by for a lifetime without regret.

Chapter 3
Prettier, Better, Stronger?

A new concept has surfaced in ethical debates: human enhancement, the improvement of human beings. This includes both efforts to model the shape of the human body as desired and approaches to optimizing cognitive capabilities such as concentration or memory or to using appropriate medications to give a gentle boost to one's emotional state. What should we think of this? This chapter critically examines the "imperative of success" that dominates our age and turns it back to the actual questions: What society do we want to live in? How much do we want to demand of ourselves and others? How can we lead a good life?

Why Do We Want to Optimize Everything?

The French existentialist philosopher Jean-Paul Sartre (1905–1980) once said, "Man is nothing other than what he makes himself." With these words Sartre described a feeling for life and a trend that has significantly intensified especially in the last few years. Biomedicine and biotechnology have produced ever more powerful methods of intervening in the human body and shaping it as we see fit. The pharmaceutical industry has made a growing palette of performance-enhancing medications available. More and more healthy people use various psychoactive and neuroactive pharmaceuticals to lift themselves up in the broadest sense or to brighten depressive moods and relieve anxieties. According to a 2009 health report by a German health insurance (DAK), 40% of the people surveyed assume that medications against memory deficits or depressions due to aging or disease can also be effective in healthy people. Every 20th person confirms having taken such medications without any medical necessity.[29] According to a current study by scientists and physicians in Mainz, Germany, even every fifth university student uses synthetic drugs to improve their performance.[30] What is happening here?

What preparations are there and what effects do they have on a healthy person?

Antidementia drugs stimulate brain metabolism and counteract the degradation of cognitive capabilities. Psychoactive drugs are used to treat chronic fatigue, anxiety, or depression as well as to increase drive. Amphetamines are effective against restlessness and nervousness.

No significant effect on the performance and mood of healthy persons has yet been demonstrated for medications with doping potential. "The increasing public interest in neuroenhancement," according to Dimitris Repantis, researcher at Berlin's Charité Medical Center, "is in remarkable contrast to the lack of evidence for enhancement effects of available psychoactive substances."[31] However, reports of personal experience mention the great subjective effect, albeit along with drastic emotional side effects and a high potential for addiction.[32]

In my opinion, we can only understand current tendencies toward perfection if we place them in the larger context of the development of modern society, when we understand them as an expression of a verdict of success under which modern life stands.

The Imperative of Success

Modern man has been released into his freedom. Today we are no longer subject to any specific conventions, but can choose, seemingly freely, our own personal values and goals to follow. A common orientation for all people seems to have become impossible so that the only unifying element that remains is the freedom to decide as one pleases. Man has been thrown back on himself and what he does with his life is up to him. This newly won freedom of being able to decide "what" to "do" with life not only increases one's personal responsibility for the result of this decision, but also casts life as something that can also "fail." Merely the idea that not only this enterprise or that one but life as a whole can fail seems to be a result of this modern freedom, insofar as from this perspective the individual ultimately bears responsibility when his life, by whatever yardstick, proves a failure. What was initially seen as a *release* from traditional obligations and from the tenets and commitments of convention reveals itself upon closer scrutiny to be a key *burden* on modern man. The apparent freedom of being able to choose one's goals in life is coupled with the imperative of making this life a success, that is, to lead it in such a way that it can appear as successful. This imperative states: be successful in leading your own life.

We are thus all more or less directly subject to a collective success postulate. We place ourselves under intense pressure to be able to present our life as a successful one. We are forced not to live life but to actively lead it in pursuit of commonly favored goals because only in this manner will we be recognized as a "full-fledged person" in an ostensibly free society. Naturally, this state of affairs is not solely attributable to the new "freedom" given to a person; rather, it is the case that the advent of the imperative of success has reduced life to an assessable "product" that can also fail. Largely dictated by a society based on consumption and performance, the modern imperatives and constraints suggest that the individual only has value as long as he makes something of himself. Thus, his value is not intrinsic in his existence but is assessed according to which "life product" he has succeeded in producing with his actions.

When the value of one's own self depends on whether one succeeds in presenting his own life as a "successful" one and when this success is primarily geared to the tenets of a performance-based society, then efficiency acquires a high value. For without the physical and emotional constitution necessary to following this "imperative of success," the individual gets the feeling of not belonging. In a society geared to being able to "do" everything, efficiency assumes the role of an enabling cause. As efficiency tends to be regarded as the only possibility for leading a good life, it becomes elevated to a social absolute, ushering in an irrational cult of competition. The media and the advertising industry accordingly proclaim a never-ending appeal to strive for efficiency, beauty, and youth and in a sense to create oneself anew with each passing day.

The larger context in which we must reflect on these tendencies is capitalism with its implicit promise of finding salvation here on earth. Yet, according to capitalist thinking, this salvation exists only if one wins the competition. And in order to win, the individual must be continuously active, grasp every opportunity, and continuously optimize himself. Nothing less is demanded of him than to be flexible in every regard, to subject himself anew to the requirements of competition with each passing day. This subjugation is referred to as "positioning" but essentially represents nothing more than the imperative to subordinate oneself. We obey it in light of the continuous threat of losing the competition. The more winning the competition becomes what we strive for, the more we sacrifice no less than our own identity, and in so doing become alienated from ourselves. We want to win and along the way we forget to be ourselves.

The "Despair of Possibility"

Added to this is the fact that we live in constant fear and make the wrong decision, in constant fear of missing something. The Danish philosopher and theologist Søren Kierkegaard (1813–1855), in his 1849 book *The Sickness unto Death*, grasped something that is particularly relevant to today's society:

> "Now if possibility outruns necessity, the self runs away from itself, so that it has no necessity whereto it is bound to return—then this is the despair of possibility." (Søren Kierkegaard)

It is in this despair of possibility that we live today. We have many more possibilities than ever before and yet we despair of them because we sense that we cannot take advantage of all of them. We have to decide in favor of one possibility and are forced to pass up many others. Thus, we live in perpetual fear of having made the wrong decision. This fear also gives us the feeling of being imperfect because we have to limit ourselves. This has to do with the fact that the possibilities available to us today do not merely represent an offer but by their very existence assume the nature of a demand. The possibilities are not without obligation but urge the person to actually take advantage of them. And this plunges a person into perpetual perplexity, driven to take advantage of as many possibilities as possible under the impression that this will lead to a fulfilled life.

But is it not the case that the opposite is true? The more we race after possibilities, the greater it seems to me is the danger of inner alienation, of emptiness. This emptiness occurs because today we are under pressure to be constantly successful. When success means exhausting all possibilities, then a person lives in a perpetual feeling of deficiency, a feeling of somehow being unsatisfactory, of somehow failing. As I see it, the aspirations of enhancement, of "optimization" in the widest sense, can only take hold because in our competitive society the whole of life is understood as a challenge to maximize, as a challenge to accumulate, and to optimally exploit possibilities. The only problem is that if we place life in the service of maximizing what is possible, what happens to us ourselves? What happens to the essence of our own personality? Maximization is merely a method of propagation, but without regard to the quality that is to be propagated. The only quality is winning the competition, but this poses the questions: Why should we win? What is the goal? At times it seems that it is all about winning today so as to be able to win even more quickly tomorrow. But what is the point of all this? And above all and once again: What happens to us ourselves? What happens to focusing on one's own being, to reflecting on what constitutes my being? The imperative of submitting to the dictate of winning ignores this self. This is the reason for the emptiness, the shell in the midst of overabundant possibilities.

I feel that we can adequately formulate the question of an ethics of enhancement, of an ethics of optimization, only in this larger context. The concept of optimization in itself postulates the existence of means that can improve the human being. Yet I ask myself: What exactly is an improvement for the human being? Should it not primarily be about the human being, in the sense of each individual one of us as a person, and about the question of what is good for him before we demand he be improved? In my eyes, the greatest weakness of the entire optimization debate lies in the view that every form of enhancing human capabilities in itself represents an improvement.

67

Increasing the effectiveness of human thought processes and enhancing cognitive recall may well represent an improvement with respect to certain goals, for example, being able to function smoothly in a performance society. But it would be shortsighted to conclude from this that the improvement in efficiency in itself is an improvement for mankind.

When one says that the goal of the human being as a human being is simply to be quicker, then it is undoubtedly good to optimize his brain functions. But is this really the goal of the human being? What exactly is a good life? Or in other words: Does the dissemination of means of optimization really lead to a better life, to a good life? There are a few things to consider here.

Endangering the Good Life

What is threatening about this development in my eyes is less the health risk from drug abuse. What is threatening is primarily this: the more popular enhancement methods become, the less acceptance there will be of those people desiring to conform less fully to a society geared to functioning. As the more things become possible, the more things are seen as intolerable. This is evident in attitudes toward children. In an age when dispensing Ritalin (a preparation that improves concentration) to children is regarded as normal, children with attention deficit disorder are increasingly seen as people who no longer must be "tolerated" because there is a medication for their condition. Willingness to accept them in their current state would be nothing less than irrational because something can be "done." For this reason, they are increasingly regarded as intolerable because the willingness to show patience toward them is decreasing. In this manner, the existence of medications like Ritalin promotes an atmosphere of intolerance.

> The medication is not merely an option; it simultaneously awakens the social expectation that people will be accordingly modulated if medications are available for their condition.

And it is not only the lack of acceptance that becomes widespread. At the same time, the expectation arises of using medications to eliminate "nonconformity" in the widest sense as quickly as possible. Other forms of therapy such as psychotherapy, family therapy, investing in relationships, or simply listening are now less accepted for the very reason that they would take effect only slowly. Quick success is preferred, although experience shows that slower success is invariably more sustainable. Giving preference to the quick fix has already become a measurable result of the widespread use of medications for psychosocial problems. This puts people in a bind; it is nearly impossible to buck the trend.

In addition to this there are numerous cases in which people must resort to using the medication to help children with attention deficit disorder. Yet at the same time, serious attention or memory deficits often are the result of family or social problems which are glossed over by taking the pills. But does it seem more reasonable in the interest of sustainability to solve social problems socially instead of simply glossing over social evils with medications (in a similar vein, see Chapter 1, p. 19)? Therapists who have a genuine interest in their patients will argue in favor of a sustainable therapy which, while requiring more time and effort, will help the entire person and not alienate him from himself.

Opportunity Becomes Constraint

A group of seven scholars from the areas of medicine, psychiatry, philosophy, and law, in addition to studying the risks and social consequences, also examined the opportunities of improved medications for the brain. In their memorandum, they come to the conclusion[33] that there are no convincing objections to pharmaceutical improvement of the brain or psyche. Advocates of enhancement essentially see this as the natural continuation of human-controlled evolution. In light of the fact that man has always made use of technologies to improve his nature, the new technologies do not represent a radical change. The ethical problems would thus essentially begin with the issue of just distribution or, respectively, equal opportunity: What consequences would it have if such preparations were made available to everyone able to pay in addition to the group of those receiving the medication as therapy? Would that not lead to a massive loss of equality of opportunity within society?

I would like to turn this question around: Would the problems resulting from the biotechnological possibilities be solved by giving everyone free access to these preparations in the future? But would this gain? If everyone dopes then everyone is more or less equal so to speak, simply on a higher level. It is like in sports: an athlete only has an advantage from doping if most of the others do not have this opportunity. What appears at first glance to be an individual advantage reveals itself on closer inspection to be a social loss because one can no longer refrain from doping without the fear of being disadvantaged. That is the paradox of this endeavor. Doping was introduced in an effort to gain an advantage from it. It was introduced to improve the individual athlete's position. The spread of the practice has transformed this positive orientation into a negative one, the fear of being at a disadvantage by refraining from doping. That means what initially arose as an opportunity to advance oneself has now become a means of protecting oneself against being disadvantaged.

> The opportunity has become a constraint and being able to win has become avoiding a disadvantage.

Analogously to this argumentation, the argument is increasingly made in connection with preimplantation genetic diagnostics (see Chapter 2, p. 46) that there is a "moral duty" to optimize (in this case the genetic makeup), namely the duty to "position the child as well as possible or at least no worse than others."[34] I call this a logic of fear arising from the logic of production.

In Praise of Forgetting

We always say it is a desirable goal not to forget anything. But is that really true? Should not the question really be: How much memory loss is really good for a person? For we can ultimately orient ourselves not only when we can retain but also and primarily when we can forget. A human being must learn to forget what is unessential. He constantly makes unconscious decisions which make him forget what is unimportant so that he can concentrate on what is essential. That is a very complex and very creative process. Thus, when I say it is a desirable goal to increase his recall, I must also specify which recall with respect to which content should be increased. For the ability to remember simply everything would impair us rather than help us as it would include all the unnecessary information we store. I am reminded of Jorge Luis Borges' famous short story "Funes the Memorious." That means the ability to remember more is only something positive for a person when he also optimizes his ability to forget. Not to mention the fact that for many people in many situations being able to forget is a blessing. Thus, it is clear that enhanced recall is not an advantage per se.

In an age characterized by an efficiency mindset, we can easily conclude that not only at work but also in personal life, whatever is quicker and more efficient is invariably better than what we achieve less quickly and only indirectly. But does not man require obstacles, detours, and resistance in order to mature? Enhancement alludes to achieving a goal without exertion. Yet this would only be good for a person if the exertion itself were merely seen as a negative circumstance with respect to the goal. Yet if we understand this having to exert oneself as an important component of our experience, then an enhancement focused solely on efficiency appears questionable. Therefore, society, but also each of us for ourselves, should consider to what extent something can have value because we learn something in the process, yet primarily because only then do we have the feeling of having produced the result ourselves, indeed because it is only through this exertion that we recognize who we are.

Is Optimization a Path to Happiness?

It is often claimed that human happiness can be attained more quickly with enhancement preparations, especially in the form of mood-altering drugs. Here, too, I would advocate taking a closer look. The study of happiness has a long tradition in philosophy. One important tradition in the attempt to define this difficult concept more precisely goes back to the ancient Greek philosopher Aristotle (384–322 BC). For him, happiness (eudaimonia) is not simply a state of wellbeing, rather an activity in which our rational action is optimally realized. Human happiness, according to Aristotle, arises when one best succeeds in living a life that realizes human virtues.

"Every art and every inquiry, and similarly every action and pursuit, is thought to aim at some good; and for this reason the good has rightly been declared to be that at which all things aim." (Aristotle, Nicomachean Ethics, translated by W. D. Ross)

Happiness for Aristotle is thus a successful life, not in the sense of the empty imperative of success to which we have to submit today, but in such a manner that the life in the world, in public, with the other person finds specific "joints to connect with." This includes a relationship between one's own actions and the outside world. The nature of happiness lies less in an internal emotional state but rather in realizing a certain form of life. Joy is nothing that one can strive for in itself. On the contrary, it simply arises when a person has the feeling that he can contribute his abilities and he succeeds in his efforts. Happiness is thus not merely a simple emotional state in the sense of wellbeing. Happiness is a way of leading life, it is life being led. From Aristotle's perspective, we could therefore say that the attempt to bring about happiness by pharmacological means misses the mark: for there can be no genuine happiness in artificially creating a virtual feeling of happiness lacking any connection to the real world. On the contrary, this would lead more to the person becoming alienated from his world and would stand in the way of his happiness rather than promoting it. Experiencing happiness requires more than the efficient manufacture of a synthetic sensation of happiness.

A person who feels happy because of the pills he takes but is in fact in a desolate situation is hardly what we would call a happy person. Happiness ultimately requires a concordance of feeling and reality.

After these objections to the unreflected acceptance of enhancement's promises of salvation, I now come to the issue that in my eyes lies at the heart of the entire optimization debate: What can we mean by a good life? Or more precisely: Is the improvement in efficiency really a path to a good life, and is the mere improvement of human capabilities actually a good goal?

Conditions for a Good Life

The enhancement methods seek to optimize the means in order to achieve a goal better or more quickly. Focusing on the means in this manner means that we can easily lose sight of the question of what is really important. Concentrating on acceleration does not only mean increasing and expanding our scope of action as is often claimed. On the contrary, focusing exclusively on efficiency narrows life to a purely economic perspective. We lead a life that rules out alternatives from the outset. By putting all our energy into efficiency and into further, higher, and faster, we become blind to all the turns and surprises that life holds in store, to the unexpected things that life has to offer. A fundamental problem of enhancement is not the acceleration as such but the fact that acceleration constricts the expanse of life in a very specific manner, that it fails to acknowledge the value of the detour and makes us blind to the sense of living a life that is fundamentally open.

Living an Open Life

My purpose is not to glorify failure, but the obstacles, the failure in specific situations, are not the catastrophes that we initially make them out to be. On the contrary, they are necessary occurrences if a person is to acquire the ability to perform great deeds and find himself. Advocating enhancement entirely ignores this aspect and suggests that the goal alone constitutes the good life. We forget that it is often the path that constitutes the purpose and not the goal alone. No one has expressed this better than the founder of existential philosophy Søren Kierkegaard, who wrote in his book *Either/Or* published in 1843:

"The great thing is not to be this or that, but to be ourselves."

This "ourselves," this success postulate, keeps cropping up. At the beginning, I elucidated how the advocates of enhancement refer back to principles such as autonomy. Their argument is that individual freedom should come to bear here. When we consider that the cultural basis for the aspirations of enhancement is ultimately the competition mindset, then we must realize that a decision for en-hancement driven purely by competition does not occur as a result of inner freedom but out of the necessity imposed by this competition. For competition will invariably lead to one thing: the obligation to submit to the rules of competition. People like to talk about autonomy in this connection, but it is basically a matter of conformity, of adapting to and ultimately internalizing the attitude that there are no alternatives to enhancement. This is doubly paradoxical when we consider that many people resort to using performance-enhancing drugs because they feel they are otherwise unable to withstand the pressure of the demands of today's society. They address their prob-lem with the methods that created the problem in the first place. The medication follows the same principles as the problem they seek to solve. Here we see that there is something paradoxical about using medications as a means to counteract the pressure to perform. That this could happen is related to the fact that competition ultimately acts as a social constraint and overshadows everything else.

Enhancement preparations promise greater autonomy but in fact only strengthen outside control and cement inequality and especially self-exploitation.

And there is something else to consider when we speak of autonomy. People forget that autonomy includes not only freedom but also authenticity. I would like to exercise my freedom in such a manner that I feel I am the actual originator of my actions. I would like to write the script of my life myself and see myself as its actual author. But how is this possible when my action must be understood as the result of taking a medication? How can one be an author while simultaneously making oneself the object of a pharmacological process by taking pills? What still originates within me when what I achieve must ultimately be attributed to the effect of a medication?

Critics often respond that drinking coffee is not viewed as self-instrumentalization either. Yet this disregards the fact that drinking coffee is not solely directed toward increasing performance but is more part of a shared culture in which the increase in performance is a more or less desirable side effect. This becomes clear when we consider that everyone would find it absurd to substitute the coffee maker in a company with a pill dispenser. For this reason, I would say that taking pills represents a certain form of self-instrumentalization where we can no longer say without question that the doped person is indeed fully the actual originator of his actions.

Preserving a Sense of What Is as It Is

To rely on enhancement means to fundamentally proceed from the premise that life is first and foremost a project, an act of building, in which the product is to be seen as the result of what we have made and actively changed. Seen from such a perspective, life is something that is not "full" but a defect that must be eliminated. Naturally, life can only succeed if we shape it and thus in the strict sense live it (and not simply be lived). It is also correct that life will be not fulfilled if we do not formulate our own goals. Then again it is still a dubious limitation to see life only as something to be shaped. Our freedom and our success do not depend on what we do but above all on whether we succeed in achieving a healthy balance between being able to do and letting be. Achieving this balance assumes that we learn not only to see life from the perspective of not yet existing and still to be done, but also to continually increase our appreciation of the sense and value of what already exists.

Our failure to acknowledge the good in givenness is one of the fundamental deficits of our age, an age primarily geared to enhancement measures. Desires for enhancement exclude insight into the value of what is given and render impossible something I feel is crucial to a successful life: the fundamental attitude of gratitude. Gratitude for what is. Gratitude for life as such. Gratitude for the smallest things which can become something special by virtue of this fundamental attitude of gratitude. Without this fundamental attitude, it would be difficult for us to find something like fulfillment because the noncompletable is a basic premise of the optimization mindset; it never reaches its goal. The more we optimize and in so doing exclude gratitude for what is given, the more we are forced onto a treadmill where there can never be enough optimization. The Greek philosopher Epicurus (341–271 BC) fittingly expressed it in these words:

"Nothing is enough for the man to whom enough is too little."

77

Today we have the tendency to believe that only what we have selected for ourselves is good because there is no longer anything that we must simply accept. But do we not overlook that fact that our entire life is permeated with determinants that we have not chosen and cannot choose? To deny these determinants would be foolish and would stand in the way of a successful life. To live a good life, one must recognize that everyone is more the result of his determinants than his own doing. Every human being is thrown into a world which he did not choose himself, which existed before him and which ultimately made him possible. He would not be here without this world which for him is simply given. Furthermore, every human being is put into a certain epoch which he also did not choose himself. For him it is simply given. Thus, the key conditions of our existence are givens and not entities we have selected.

Modern man lives under the assumption of shaping his destiny himself and of being able to be or having to be his own creator. This perspective of radical openness blocks our view of ourselves because it sees in people only what is open and shapable and it leaves no room for recognizing what was already there in such and such a manner. This leads to a situation in which our energy is occasionally focused excessively on this illusory goal of eliminating what is given. This threatens to squander the potential that lies in accepting what is given and with it one's own being and learning how best to cope with it. The German philosopher and essayist Hans Blumenberg (1920–1996) put it in a nutshell when he emphasized that in the modern world "nothing that is, must be." Yet this "that is" has a value, and that is something we must consider again when we claim to have understood the deep ramifications of the optimization of human beings as the collective wish of our age.

What am I trying to say here? My intention is not to advocate a return to an unconditional acceptance of fate. That would be foolish and would not do justice to man as a being endowed with the power of reason. Our problematic attitude toward fate does not begin where we struggle against fate but only begins where it is suggested that modern man no longer needs to accept fate because medicine can give him absolute freedom to shape his body himself, the freedom to select his progeny himself (see Chapter 2), and the freedom to "optimize" himself as he sees fit. The implicit promise of these absolute freedoms is the real problem of many areas of glamorous modern medicine.

For this is illusory! Indeed, it is not freedom when, for example, aesthetic medicine suggests one could select one's own body. Because this allegedly being able to select for oneself has brought with it a new lack of freedom, namely that maybe as soon as tomorrow this self-selected body shape will have to be tested for its suitability to the goals associated with it. If the body is no longer fate but only the result of a person's own choice as many areas of aesthetic medicine suggest, then this being able to choose has given rise to a new lack of freedom, because now a person can also be made responsible for what has been chosen and will have to question it anew with each passing day. The moment we substitute what is given with something of our own choice, we enter a spiral of continually having to choose again, a spiral of constant comparison. Gone is the carefree spirit in which we once dealt with our own self.

In this setting, I advocate a new insight into the need for limits to what is feasible. Ultimately, it is a matter of being able to accept limits, but above all of being able to accept oneself.

In our society and also as individuals, we now tend to react to the world with the attitude of desire and are neglecting to pause and to be content, and we are losing a sense of proportion. At the same time, we know from ancient philosophy that no one can be happy without the cardinal virtue of a sense of proportion. What we lack most is a sense of proportion in dealing with desire! Modern man desires to be the very beginning of everything, to live a life without flaws and not to have to put up with anything. The philosopher Martin Heidegger called this the "will to will." And it is precisely this "will to will" in our attitude of entitlement that ultimately makes us unhappy, fearful, and even despairing. We fall victim to our claims of being able to make the world and fail to see that in reality our happiness lies in ourselves, specifically in the inner attitude with which we encounter the world.

An inner attitude that could tell us that the feeling of satisfaction with the world cannot be produced with a pill. An attitude that tells us that the good life cannot consist in merely functioning better but in experiencing a feeling of richness as an entire person. And this richness includes avoiding premature "closing" and wanting to reduce the entirety of life to certain qualities. This richness includes being open to the expanse of life and refusing all types of entrapments. I would even go so far as to say to remain open for what is unsolicited, for what we do not choose ourselves. For what is valuable in life is often what we have not planned, that which simply occurs, as long as we remain open for the new event. Therefore, I would conclude that the happy life does not consist in achieving a perfect life but in taking a stand against paralysis at every turn.

Thus, it is our attitude that tells us man's alleged imperfections, his performance limits, his vulnerability, have a deeper significance. Maybe this inner attitude can lead to our appreciating what is imperfect and not only what is seemingly perfect. To an appreciation of the imperfect, not in the sense of denying its drawbacks, but in the sense of an attitude of humility in the acceptance of that which could be perfect. For we really do not know at all what the perfect human being should be. Therefore, it should be a matter of creating good social conditions for the imperfect human being instead of forcing him to become ostensibly perfect only to adapt to the imperfect conditions of the modern performance society.

Strengthening Resolve Instead of Promoting Conformity

My criticism is not intended as a blanket condemnation of every enhancement for every person at every time. On the contrary, my aim is to draw attention to a general tendency rather than to dismiss it categorically. I simply suggest we consider that optimization tendencies, although they can be seamlessly integrated into the positive notions of efficiency and control we propagate, can ultimately become questionable if they are affirmed and reinforced without reflection. However, this does not rule out the use of these approaches in specific cases where it may appear advisable or at least tolerable. There will be situations in which the desire for enhancement arises from distress and where no other help is available. Nonetheless, my critical reflection is intended to open up a perspective that even in this specific case helps us to become aware of the goals associated with enhancement: Might they not be of questionable value? Do they actually deliver what I envision? Or will I unintentionally become caught in a spiral that leads far away from me? Criticizing the values of enhancement does not necessarily lead to a paternalistic, patronizing attitude. As criticism it can also give the person willing to undergo enhancement the ability to appreciate every facet of his desire.

When therapists are willing to comply without thinking with what is usually a very abstract self-optimization, then they aid and abet the fundamental notions I have described; in a certain sense they become accomplices of these notions, accomplices of an economic society geared solely to performance and efficiency. Acceptance of the goals of efficiency, speed, and control by the health care professions stabilizes and confirms these values. To be aware of this can be in the interest of the person expressing a desire for neuroenhancement. We have seen how social trends can exert pressure on the individual and how he often can hardly escape this pressure, although doing exactly that is correct and important in order for him to find himself. Particularly in the case of people who resort to using doping medications due to a lack of self-confidence, this raises the question of whether appropriate help on the part of the health care professions would consist in treating the underlying lack of self-confidence rather than the symptoms (see later).

In addition to this, we must always bear in mind that medicine can also squander its trust as an institution dedicated to the person seeking help if it prescribes doping medications whenever they are desired. The more this is done without reflection, the closer medicine moves toward becoming a simple service provider that in my opinion has little to do with the art of healing. Whereas prescribing neuro-enhancers can indeed help the individual patient in certain cases, their widespread application without reflection can turn this individual help into a collective pressure to conform. For this reason, the responsibility of the therapist becomes particularly important, as the therapist should follow only the individual's best interests and not market criteria.

A therapeutic ethos that only offers a pill in response to many people's fear of being left behind by a performance society does not really do justice to the patient. Should it not also be part of an "ethics of therapy" that the therapist does not unthinkingly fulfill desires but always attempts to encounter the individual with a fundamental attitude of wanting to help? That can occasionally be the medication, yet it should always initially begin with entering into a relationship with the patient borne not by prescriptions but by understanding.

In the debate about the optimization of human beings, we tend to focus too much on a single characteristic, while losing sight of the whole picture. For me, it is about developing a holistic view of this problem; it is about the entire person, not just one characteristic. I feel that a human being cannot become happy merely by functioning better but that he is dependent on living with the feeling that his intrinsic value is grounded not in his efficiency but in his very being, in his being able to be as he is. The more we lose this feeling, the more we fall victim to self-alienation. We then tend to regard our own body only as an instrument with which we can achieve (or fail to achieve) socially accepted goals. Modern man uses his body as a tool, forgetting that in this manner he simply allows himself to be entrapped by the collective expectations.

When we speak of therapeutic help for people who request the doctor to prescribe such pills, we must realize that help in such cases can also mean rekindling an awareness that they do not need artificial performance enhancement in the form of doping pills in order to feel that they have value. Maybe such therapies should be geared to strengthening people's resolve to make them immune to the temptation of using doping drugs to conform completely.

Taking this thought to its logical conclusion, maybe good medicine in the sense of the art of healing is medicine that itself shows resolve and does not act as a vehicle for each and every goal of a performance society ruled by economics.

In short, it can be said that we live in a society that gives people the task of being perfect. Yet the more perfect a person becomes, the more deficient he becomes. Striving for perfection in the sense of absolute intolerance to flaws can become a regular obsession. We lose sight of what is really important. This suggests that the drive toward perfection is only a desperate attempt on the part of modern man to replace meaning lost in the course of secularization and the increasing use of technology by obsessively clinging to the ideal of perfection. The delusion of perfection could then be understood as a response to the lack of transcendence in a market society geared exclusively to efficiency.

Modern society focuses solely on feasibility and uses technology and science to determine consummation on the basis of perfection. This experiment is doomed to fail. We have seen that the mindset of technological progress cannot be the sole measure of a good life. This narrowing to functionality and suitability leads to an attitude in which there are only standardized concepts of perception: people who must all achieve the same high-performance goals and are all expected to function constantly. Yet the actual consummation of man lies not in his efficiency but in his uniqueness. Every human being is perfect because he is distinctive. In this sense, our technological striving for perfection becomes blindness to forms of perfection that already exist and cannot be produced. It is the distinctive brilliance of life itself.

Therefore, it is important that medicine gain new perspectives of the human being, that it open approaches in which, despite all the striving for control, awe is not forgotten and which allow something like euphoria in the face of the variety of human and nonhuman life on earth. Medicine's striving to exceed limits and to seize, subjugate, and control what exists has undoubtedly brought many blessings to mankind. Yet when it is reduced to this seizing, without pairing this striving with a fundamental attitude of humility and respect for what is, then medicine will bring forth a fundamental attitude that will ultimately turn against life itself. The value and the richness of life do not lie in what can be measured and increased, but in life itself. And the more we can free ourselves from the one-sided categories of performance of our age, the more we can learn a new tranquility, then the more we will recognize what is really important in life and in so doing be able to become happy.

Chapter 4
Is Health a Duty?

We live in a society in which health is regarded as the highest good—from the perspective of both the individual and the population as a whole. Health today is no longer part of medicine but is increasingly becoming an important economic factor. Empowerment is the new concept: activation of the individual to assume personal responsibility, while the state simultaneously withdraws from its duty to provide for the public welfare. Yet what are the limits and what are the drawbacks when we increasingly bear responsibility for our health ourselves? This chapter raises objection to the insidious notion of sickness as "guilt" and shows that personal responsibility only functions when it is anchored in social responsibility. A healthy person is not one without impairments but one who learns how to cope creatively with his own limitation and his fundamental vulnerability.

Personal Responsibility Is the New Paradigm

The passive patient who consults the expert, the doctor, and is told what to do has become obsolete—at least in political platforms. The guiding principle today is the active patient as an expression of the engaged citizen, one who does not merely follow the doctor's orders but who sees himself as an expert on his own physical and emotional constitution, contributes accordingly, and makes decisions on his own responsibility. As his own responsibility increases, the patient is redefined as a user, an active player, who on his own initiative obtains the pertinent information and explores the options necessary for managing his health impairment. Not only does he utilize the advice and assistance of the physician, but he also consults other professionals—psychologists, pharmacists, or experts from health insurance providers, self-help groups, and experts from consumer protection associations. The modern patient assumes responsibility for his health himself and makes use of the physician and other health advisors largely as he sees fit.

"Health Literacy"

"Improving the health literacy" of the patients becomes particularly important in this setting. The World Health Organization (WHO) and the European Union (EU) have defined health literacy as the "individual's ability" to "take decisions in daily life that have a positive effect on health." "Health literacy," it continues, "makes people capable of self-determination and of accepting the freedom to arrange and decide with respect to their health. It improves the ability to find and understand health information and accept responsibility for one's own health."

Health literacy is thus a concept that explicitly rejects a patronizing health education. It replaces the previous health education, which was primarily geared to avoiding risks, with the emphasis on the competence of each individual. The aim is not primarily to ingrain certain changes in behavior in order to avoid disease but to mobilize one's own strengths. Thus, this conception relies on motivating a person to control his own behavior. This is referred to as empowerment. The goal of health education would accordingly be to include the world in which the patient lives as well as strengthening his individual problem-solving abilities.

According to Ilona Kickbusch's definition, health literacy can be divided into five areas:

- *Competence in personal health.*
- *Competence in system orientation, meaning navigating the health care system.*
- *Competence in "consumer behavior," meaning the ability to make "service decisions."*
- *Competence in the workplace setting, meaning the ability to avoid accidents and occupational diseases.*
- *Finally, competence in health care policy, meaning the ability to become engaged for patient rights and other health-related issues.*[35]

This list unmistakably illustrates that health literacy, reflecting the modern aspirations, applies less to the patient in the classic sense than to the user, the "consumer." It is he who should become empowered as soon as possible, meaning put in the position of being able to autonomously assume responsibility for himself. Yet it also becomes clear that health literacy is not simply a matter of acquiring certain knowledge. Rather, at its core, it is the ability to make many important decisions oneself, including those related to issues of one's own health, and to acquire a certain practical competence in dealing with these questions. Thus, in discussing in health literacy, it is helpful not only to limit ourselves to only the five areas of competence mentioned— personal health, navigating the health care system, consumer behavior, health care policy, and the workplace setting—but also to differentiate three separate levels of health literacy:

- *Functional competence, referring to the ability to acquire simple information (essentially the ability to read and understand texts).*

- *Interactive competence, examining and interpreting this information in a communicative exchange with other people.*
- *Critical competence as the ability to question information as well.*[36]

Promote and Demand

Naturally, all these goals and aspirations are to be welcomed. Who would not like to determine himself how he deals with health? It is obvious that people do not want to be patronized by experts, and it is a great gain that the old paternalism in which the doctor simply dictated to the patient what he had to do has since disappeared at least from political platforms. Yet it is important to see the modern concept of health literacy in the context in which it was formulated. For health literacy is not simply formulated as a goal in a vacuum but in the context of a new understanding of the state and society. It is formulated at a time when the welfare state, whose duty is to ensure that health care is provided to the population, has been declared obsolete and the call to modernize it is becoming ever louder. What is now called for is for the "activating state." The modern understanding of the welfare state is based less on providing for citizens than on the concept of personal responsibility. The premise of the political system is thus to promote the citizen's competences with the ultimate goal of obligating the citizen while simultaneously releasing the state from those obligations. While the welfare state must purportedly be maintained at all costs, it is in fact being dismantled behind the facade of euphemistic concepts such as freedom of choice, engagement, and personal responsibility.

It is not uninteresting to note that the state's imposition of an obligation to assume responsibility has been coupled with the rhetoric of emancipation, of liberation from patronization.[37] This represents an ingenious twofold strategy. The citizen is to be provided by the state with all the prerequisites for individual success while the state can withdraw from its obligations. We could aptly summarize under the slogan "promote and demand." The first step is to encourage individual competences with respect to personal health behavior. If this does not suffice, then the second step is to threaten sanctions. But are we not overlooking the fact that the acceptance of responsibility must be linked to certain basic requirements? In other words, must people not first be rendered able to assume responsibility before they are threatened with sanctions? I think it is important to take a closer look here.

The Limits of Personal Responsibility

With the concept of personal responsibility, I feel we forget all too easily that those segments of the population that statistically bear the greatest risk of becoming sick are on average also least able to take health promotion into account in their behavior. Due perhaps to their social status, they often simply have no choice and have neither the financial means nor the freedom of choice that is present to a greater extent among the higher social strata. This means nothing less than that one first must be able to afford health-promoting behavior! The term "prevention paradox" has been introduced to describe this situation. In essence, efforts at prevention approach often fail to produce results because they generally reach those people first who need prevention the least. Conversely, the emphasis on personal responsibility further disadvantages those who are already disadvantaged. This shows that with the pathos of patient competence and personal responsibility we fail to reach precisely the people who would have a vital interest in maintaining or improving health. Here, emphasizing personal responsibility is a strategy that is too one-sided because these people do not lack the enlightenment or good will, rather the inner resources and in particular favorable structural conditions.

In this setting, I find the increasing demolition of social welfare today extremely problematic. The more we reduce social safeguards, the more we rob the already underprivileged social strata of the chance to become individually responsible. The reason why the system is nonetheless structured this way is that we have internalized the economic mindset to such an extent that we no longer notice how greatly it has altered our understanding of justice.

> What is now occurring must be described as a shift away from justice based on need toward justice based on merit.

Yet most things in life are not the result of our own failings. In other words, there are social disadvantages that must be first equalized before we can even assume a justice of performance. Today we only look at the fact that in theory no one is denied access to social benefits, yet we fail to recognize that the starting conditions for this competition vary greatly. Under the undifferentiated paradigm of personal responsibility, we are thus on the verge of splitting society into two parts, into laudable healthy people and sick people who deserve sanctions.

We must remember that belonging to a certain social stratum is not the only factor that determines the ability to accept personal responsibility but that all this also depends on a person's age and state of health. That means that socially disadvantaged people as well as older people and especially sick people have less of an opportunity to attain health literacy. This also has to do with the fact that these groups simply have more difficulty not only understanding information but also communicating about health maintenance issues with other people (experts, family members, self-help groups, etc.) and in communicating with them coming to realize what is important for themselves. Health literacy thus has to do not only with the ability and willingness to read but also primarily with whether a person has reliable social contacts. This is what the "interactive competence" mentioned earlier ultimately refers to. Therefore, relationship structures and not mere reading ability determine whether a person has the ability to develop health literacy.

When we bear in mind that sick people in particular have difficulty acquiring the required health literacy because they have fewer opportunities to communicate with other people, then it becomes clear that this is where we must begin. Promoting health literacy means not only supporting socially disadvantaged groups but also making an effort to include old and sick people. Yet then it immediately becomes clear that the concept of the "user" or "consumer" of health care services that is currently in fashion represents the wrong paradigm. That is also the greatest weakness of the idea of personal responsibility: it is based on the self-reliant consumer. This is precisely where the activating user concept has its limits. The patient in his role as a sick person is not first and foremost a self-reliant user of services. On the contrary, he is in a fundamentally asymmetrical position because he is dependent. In contrast to the consumer, he as a patient has no choice. He did not choose his illness and cannot choose freely among nonessential goods. He is simply dependent on them. What he needs is not first and foremost freedom of choice but simply someone who will help him. When a person becomes sick, he is initially characterized by helplessness, confusion, and lack of orientation. That does not mean that his freedom should not be absolutely respected! But in order to return to a state in which he is able to decide freely, he first needs someone who feels sympathy for him, who empathizes, who understands him, and who is willing to care for him. Only afterward can we think about empowerment.

Is Sickness Guilt?

Not only medical guides but increasingly doctors' practices and clinics as well convey the impression that health is something that one can be certain of achieving with sufficient effort and investment. In other words, it is a service that can be planned on. The healthy body is seen as evidence that one has worked hard enough on oneself.[38]

> We regard health and sickness increasingly less as fate or coincidence and increasingly more as the result of our own actions, indeed as the product of our own will.

Conversely, becoming sick is then seen as something that results from a lack of health literacy in the sense of insufficient investment in one's own health. Regardless of whether this applies to a question of lifestyle or insufficient "prophylactic screening," whoever becomes sick finds himself, in light of his obligation to assume personal responsibility, confronted with the thinly veiled accusation that the sickness is his "own fault."

The Berlin psychotherapist and health trainer Irmhild Harbach-Dietz, who herself had to learn to cope with a diagnosis of cancer, writes in her essay "Cancer and the Question of Guilt":

> "Contracting cancer as a consequence of misconduct? As for me personally, what kept going through my mind in the initial period after the

diagnosis of cancer were sentences like 'You blew it!' 'You've thrown your life out the window!' Only later did it occur to me what arrogance lies behind this way of thinking. By this logic it would mean: if I do everything right then I can't get sick—what an omnipotent notion! With such thoughts of omnipotence we forget or deny that sickness is part of life."[39]

Individualize Health Risks?

The opinion that we completely control our health and that illness is willingly "avoidable" is a mistaken assumption. Health is not an individual personality trait but depends on a structural framework and not solely on the individual. Here the perspective of responsibility has clearly been overstretched and has led to the problematic shifting of responsibility for social and structural deficits back to the individual. This has enormous repercussions for the image of the sick person and for the image of medicine. Making personal responsibility the central paradigm means seeing a person in need of help unavoidably confronted with the question of why this finding could not have been avoided with appropriate prophylactic screening. And naturally everyone would have attempted to prevent such a finding with their behavior if possible. When we elevate personal responsibility to the prevailing paradigm, then more than that will occur.

Then we withdraw our confidence from the sick person. The more personal responsibility becomes the guiding principle, the more each patient will fall under a sort of general suspicion. This can lead to a situation in which a person who has become sick is ultimately regarded as a "potential offender." And the more we would then like to go so far as to penalize this patient with sanctions should he not behave in a manner conducive to the maintenance of health, the more we maneuver him into isolation.

> We are turning a person in need of help into someone who has "violated a standard" and in so doing are doubly stigmatizing the sick person.

I find such a development highly problematic! For in this way we completely lose sight of the fact that sickness is a state of distress that first and foremost requires help and not punishment. If we view the sickness solely as a consequence of insufficient personal responsibility, then the sick person will experience it as failure and guilt. Sickness is increasingly becoming an abnormality of one's own making and moving ever closer to being cast as a character flaw. Today we tend to hold the individual almost solely responsible because this fits the prevailing credo of our age: every man is the architect of his own fortune —and every man is not only his own entrepreneur, but also his own health manager.

Just as health does not merely represent a service, sickness should not be associated with concepts such as guilt and punishment. In so doing, we would introduce a fundamental and unjustified breakdown of solidarity. On the contrary, we should focus on creating positive incentives without simultaneously signaling that we would like to distance ourselves from the person who has fallen sick. In other words, it is a matter of motivating and not of threatening punishment. Therefore, there is a big difference between whether we start a prevention campaign to *promote* health or whether we start one to *demand* health. There is a thin line between promoting and demanding, and not only in terms of semantics. A society that demands health will further cement the social divisions in that society. The privileged have sufficient resources to behave in a manner corresponding to the ideal of a health society geared to performance. Those groups in society who are already disadvantaged will be left even further behind because of their far fewer resources. Therefore, I advocate a system whereby the political system is not allowed to simply withdraw and declare the individual solely responsible for his health. The political system must also ensure that the emphasis on personal responsibility, which in itself is correct, does not gradually mutate to a demand for health armed with sanctions. Even if we subscribe to the technophilic belief in the ideal health behavior, it is very difficult to define health clearly and with it health-promoting behavior. This is due in no small measure to the interdependence of individual behavior and social conditions. The political system can easily formulate negative appeals like "Don't smoke!" and "Don't drink!" but it gets harder when it comes to determining positive behavior. The notion that health is a positively definable, individually attainable achievement and can be made a duty is in my opinion a mistaken assumption. The author Juli Zeh depicted the possible consequences of such a "health dictatorship" in her novel *Corpus Delicti* (2009).

Trust in the Social Bond

The concept of activating the patient can be rather inappropriate in the case of an acute illness. Certainly, there are patients who immediately regain their orientation and can be appropriately "empowered." But many patients must first be recognized as sick people in their distress, as people who are suffering and in their suffering are allowed to feel "weak" without having health care pro-fessionals of all people admonish them to be active. Only when we give the sick person the freedom to be a patient in the original sense of the word (from the Latin "patiens" meaning patient, enduring, suffering) can we express the hope that he will find his way back to the new engagement and will again be receptive to activation. However, under no circumstances should the concept of health literacy in the sense of activation and personal responsibility be applied indiscriminately to all people as an overriding paradigm.

In other words, personal responsibility is correct and important but it only works when it is linked to joint responsibility and thus to an orientation toward the common good. We can only learn individually responsible behavior when we have first learned to trust, specifically to trust in the fact that society stands in solidarity with us, that it needs us and acts as our advocate due to a deep conviction. The more it is suggested to us via the personal responsibility paradigm that we may have forfeited our right to help, the more we will be genuinely discouraged and will withdraw. One example: What will pathologically obese people think and especially feel when they constantly hear in the media that obesity represents a huge financial burden for society? And when the emphasis on personal responsibility surreptitiously transmits the misconception that it is primarily due to a lack of will? These people are not being motivated to take individually responsible action. Thoroughly discouraged, they are cast into frustration or even depression.

Being able to accept personal responsibility requires positive motivation. It requires the basic feeling that it is worthwhile to live in this society, that is one can rely on one's environment. Personal responsibility can only take root where it is supported by a feeling of shared responsibility. Without such a feeling, any sprouting seed of personal responsibility will wither. Figuratively speaking, I see personal responsibility as a blossom that can bloom as long as the stem of the personality is well cared for. Individual responsibility is the harvest that one can reap when one has first given the entire person confidence, self-esteem, and inner strength.

Health Literacy Is More Attitude than Knowledge

Competence in the sense of strengthening the patient's autonomy is something that must first be learned. This goes beyond the mere accessibility and processing of information and primarily has to do with fundamental attitudes: How can I face changes? Am I able to experience myself as dependent without seeing this as a loss of my self-determination? I am convinced that a person can only be competent when he has learned to be so adept at coping with his illness that he no longer insists on complete restoration of his ability to function and can become so accustomed to what is irreversible that he can discover his own creative potential even in sickness. This includes the ability to experience having become sick not as an affront and the dependency on others not as the end of one's own per-spectives. Sick people achieve the best competence when they are not only "activated" but when they receive so much assistance and support that they are able to learn to live well with their illness.

Time and again, I see that severely ill patients in particular, for example, cancer patients, tend to trust their doctor's judgment and delegate their decisions to their doctor. Here, as in so many other places, one must recognize that one cannot lump all people together and that it is not simply a matter of writing informative brochures about certain medical findings and then leaving the patients alone with these brochures. One only does justice to the patient when one also feels responsibility as a physician. Patients have a personal responsibility but overemphasizing this responsibility could tempt the health care professions to neglect their own responsibility as helping professions. This would be the result of the cult of personal responsibility: that in this way all responsibility would rest on the individual and the health care professions themselves would no longer genuinely internalize their own professional responsibility. "'Responsibility' is a scarce good," notes the Frankfurt sociologist Helmut Dubiel, who himself contracted Parkinson's disease at the age of 46, in his book *Deep in the Brain* which arose from his struggle with the disease. "It cannot be placed on someone without taking it away somewhere else." The overstretched responsibility of the individual, as he indicates, could have "its downside in the new 'irresponsibility' of institutions such as the state and the health insurance and health care system that has found its way into all hypermodern societies in recent decades."[40] Especially in the face of the insidious advent of structural irresponsibilities, physicians and patients should learn to see each other as partners.

Competence in Dealing with Limitations

What do freedom and responsibility mean and what does health literacy mean in this setting? For the person who has become sick, it means that the appeal for personal responsibility must never mean simply leaving him to his fate. On the contrary, I feel that all the health care professions must unmistakably show their willingness to assume responsibility for their patients. And society should not be allowed to withdraw from its responsibility to those in distress but should do everything in its power to be alert to any hasty overextension of the activation model. Additionally and not least, this means recognizing that the state with its concentration solely on activation and personal responsibility is secretly submitting to the classic laws of the market and has assumed a market-economy mindset that can have catastrophic effects for sick people in particular.

For the healthy person, health literacy could mean not pursuing the ideal of complete wellbeing but learning to live with the limits. It could mean not feeling powerless but realizing even in a precarious situation and under poor initial conditions that every one of us has potential. Using this potential does not depend solely on money but also on the inner attitude, on the feeling of being able to find joy simply in the fact of one's existence. The French physician and philosopher Georges Canguilhem (1904–1995) defined health in this sense as a sort of safety reserve of response options:

> "The healthy person measures his health by the ability to survive the crises of his body and establish a new order."

I think health is not a state characterized by the absence of disease but one in which the disease risks and disease conditions can be taken into account as an integral part of life. Therefore, I would advocate describing health as a person's ability to behave toward his limitations and even functional disabilities in such a manner that they can be integrated into his own concept of life. A healthy person is not one without impairments but one who has found out how to cope creatively with his own limitation and his fundamental vulnerability. A healthy person would therefore be someone who is not determined exclusively by his disease and who does not see himself as powerless even if not everything "functions" equally well. Viktor von Weizsäcker (1886–1957), the German physician and founder of psychosomatic medicine, put it very succinctly when he said: "The secret of health is not capital that one can exhaust, rather it is only present where it is produced at every moment of life."

We live in a society where health is highly prized, yet it would be tragic if people did not realize that they can live a full life even in the presence of functional limitations insofar as they succeed in reflecting on their inner potential to overcome these functional limitations. In any case, it is of paramount importance that we realize that health is nothing that we can simply make or be certain of keeping with good will alone. Health is ultimately a gift that we receive without having earned and that we therefore should protect joyfully, maybe even thankfully, every day.

Personal Responsibility through Care

And what does that mean for medicine? Medicine has long based its self-image on the unshakable ethos of being on the patient's side and offering him help without question. This unquestionable aspect of helping has been the basis for the trust in the humanity of medicine. Indeed, it is what has made all of medicine appear as a guarantor of humanity.[41] Today, this unquestionable aspect of helping is gradually being rescinded, and this is being done very subtly. For this reason, physicians must unmistakably show that they will never withdraw from their core task, which consists in giving patients the indissoluble commitment that they as patients need: you will not be abandoned! Only in the deep awareness that medicine is on the side of the patient without reservation will patients feel strengthened and able to do something for their health.

Thus, the greatest danger of an excessive cult of personal responsibility lies in the fact that our society could be tempted to give up a social achievement with reference to the responsibility of the individual, namely the achievement of solidarity. A too one-sided pathos of personal responsibility could ultimately lead to erosion of public spirit, the collapse of the binding forces within our society, and the breakdown of a sense of community among all people. Each of us can only act autonomously when he feels supported by the reliability of social bonds, when he knows he has a stable frame of reference. The cult of personal responsibility has rendered this community-oriented frame of reference increasingly fragile and forces many people into an atmosphere of intimidation and fear, namely the fear of social indifference. Fear and intimidation are not a good basis for motivating people to take individually responsible action. Therefore, the concept of activation and individual responsibility must be pursued with a sense of proportion. It must not be so overstretched that what is basically a good idea ultimately leads to disastrous consequences, namely to social disintegration. Today there are shared values that cannot be framed in the entrepreneur's slogan for himself. There are values that go beyond the value of personal economic success. And the awareness of solidarity with those who are worse off is such an incalculable value. I am profoundly convinced of this!

The current era of economization, individualization, and ebbing solidarity is a great challenge for the social character of medicine because it is to be feared that medicine has fundamentally changed and moved away from its genuine social task of helping to mutate from a helper into a judge over the patient. Helping the patient attain a health-promoting way of life remains a key requirement of medicine. Yet at the same time we should maintain the awareness that medical aid for sick people must not be linked to the discussion of possible personal guilt—even in the occasional case where it may appear obvious. For good reason, the physician's actions have always been guided by the ideal of the unconditional helper. Attempts to weaken this paradigm shake the very foundations of medicine as a social practice.

For medicine to remain the patient's advocate, it also needs a framework that allows it to invest in relationships with the patient without immediately having to produce evidence that this investing in relationships has directly paid off. The investment in promoting personal responsibility through the relationship with the patient is a golden investment in the future and should also be respected by the system as a value in itself even in the absence of an immediate expected return. It is this relationship with the patient that offers the opportunity of engendering a capacity for responsibility, a capacity that can only ripen into personal responsibility with social support. Therefore, the ethical motto for the future is: not personal responsibility instead of care, but personal responsibility through care! And medicine has no greater commitment than to this unconditional care for the person in need.

Chapter 5
The Crisis of Confidence in Organ Donation

The recent disclosure of various fraud scandals has obscured the fact that transplantation medicine pursues a humane goal in its basic intention. The mistrust this has caused cannot simply be addressed by stepping up monitoring or issuing moral appeals. Instead, what needs to be done is to establish behavior that inspires confidence throughout the entire system. This means taking the worries, fears, and needs of everybody involved seriously as well as dealing frankly with the criterion of brain death and establishing a culture of mourning and parting. For organ donation is not simply a purely technological process but ultimately an act within a relationship—a relationship between one person who donates and another who receives in deep gratitude.

In October 2012, an examination commission of the German Medical Association found that there had been systematic violations of the guidelines of transplantation medicine in four of Germany's 24 liver transplantation centers in the years 2010 and 2011. Donor organs were not made available according to medical necessity and urgency, and physicians falsified patient data to give certain patients priority for donor livers. The public reacted extremely sensitively to this fraud scandal: the number of organ donations dropped 13% to the lowest level since 2002. This reaction is understandable: people only want to donate their organs when they can trust the people as well as the system blindly. Yet, on the other hand, the media treatment of this unacceptable misconduct on the part of certain physicians was so sensationalized and indiscriminate that ultimately everyone involved in transplantation medicine was branded as a potential swindler and a truly enlightened discussion hardly took place at all.

Instead, numerous suggestions were made with respect to introducing controls. Controls are undoubtedly important, although we should not succumb to the illusion that controls alone will be enough to regain the public's fundamental trust. They only ensure certainty. While certainty is essential, it alone cannot establish trust. Trust means that people are prepared to assume good motives even when they can be neither verified nor guaranteed. That is the crux of the matter in this debate! There is a lot of talk about trust, but instead of trust, the contract has been chosen as the solution, the contractual agreement to abide by this rule and that. Naturally, it is essential to abide by rules but transplantation medicine has hardly demonstrated its trustworthiness by merely following rules. Trust is created not only by following rules. Trust focuses primarily on the motivation, the fundamental attitude, the personality, and the daily routine. Therefore, the greatest challenge of the current crisis of confidence in transplantation medicine lies not in establishing control over behavior but in establishing a culture of behavior toward this topic that must engender trust and include more than just stricter control.

Conditions for Confidence

To start with, the manipulation of data as was done by various physicians is indisputably an individual violation that must be punished. Yet it should not be left at the individual level because the problem goes deeper than the recourse to a personal violation would have us believe.

Upon closer examination, we find a systemic problem in that those who operate frequently are rewarded. As a result, frequent transplantations become a must and even a question of institutional survival. This gives rise to a climate in which a few people lacking strength of character become swindlers.

Eliminate False Incentives

Therefore, I feel that punishing a few individuals is not sufficient; rather we should rethink the whole system. It is a system that is geared too much to internal competition, defines minimum quantities, creates incentives to increase the number of transplantations, and even links physicians' remuneration to the number of operations. Precisely, these incentives are detrimental and extremely dangerous. They are detrimental because they tempt physicians to depart from a purely medical perspective and give increasingly greater consideration to nonmedical goals such as their own interests in profit or prestige.

> Trust is not created merely by punishing individuals but first and foremost by critically rethinking the system of "transplantation medicine."

Physicians must not be tempted by the system itself to apply other than purely medical criteria in making decisions. Thus, I strictly oppose bonuses based on nonmedical criteria. Increasing the number of cases does not represent a purely medical goal either, rather an economic one. A medical goal, on the other hand, would be to increase the quality of treatment, here meaning quality that has a long-term effect. Offering more money for more operations in employment contracts ultimately means nothing else than that the employer assumes the physician is fundamentally corruptible and that his decision as to what treatment is indicated can be controlled by the fee offered to him.

Worries and Fears Must Be Taken Seriously

A second confidence-building aspect is the requirement of clarification and transparency. "Transparency" is not achieved simply by disclosing all figures and mapping all processes. And this is important. Even more important is that the public sense that their questions, worries, and fears are genuinely taken seriously. In this context, I feel it is important to remember that while the crisis of confidence has intensified as a result of the fraud scandals, the willingness of Germans to donate has always been rather low compared with the rest of Europe in spite of the obvious good purpose. That is exactly the reason the new law was originally introduced.

> On November 1, 2012, the German "Law Regulating the Decision Solution in the Transplantation Law" came into effect. Now the statutory and private health insurance funds regularly send letters to all insured persons above the age of 16 asking whether they want to donate organs in the case of their brain death. The goal of increasing willingness to donate organs in Germany has thus become law. The law "provides for broad education of the public on the opportunities for organ and tissue donation" (www.bmg.bund.de).

We are making it too easy for ourselves if we think that people are merely too lazy to fill out the organ donor ID. On the contrary, this is an expression of a fundamental attitude of hesitation, doubt, uncertainty, and a basic lack of trust on the part of many people. Now we are attempting to remedy this by launching moral appeals. At first glance, that seems plausible and quite reasonable. Yet such appeals are poison for a relationship of trust. An appeal implies that we should have a guilty conscience if we do not donate. It implies that it is not a personal decision because the moral appeal in itself defines which decision is "right." This suggests a clarity that makes a person feel even more uneasy and pressured. We can also imagine this as a real-life situation. If a person were in doubt as to whether he should do another person a favor and that person began to give him a guilty conscience in the event he should refuse the request, then the doubting person would withdraw and refuse the request all the more decidedly. Therefore, it would be far more appropriate to talk to the hesitating person about his hesitation, to clarify where his uncertainty lies and how it might be able to be resolved.

Citing people in poor health who could be helped by a donor organ has an emotional impact but cannot resolve the inner conflict. At best it traps a person but it does not lead to a decision that has matured in due deliberation. The trap begins with the selected terminology. The media repeatedly refers to patients waiting for an organ. And it is repeatedly emphasized that these patients must die because there are not enough donors. Yet this stylized causal relationship does not follow logically. The patients do not die of the lack of an organ but of their underlying disease. That is a big difference. And when we construct such a causal relationship it means nothing other than that organ donations are implicitly expected and that it is normal to donate. The death of a person on the waiting list is not interpreted as a natural death due to a severe disease but as the effect of insufficient willingness to donate organs. At what point can we ever speak of "insufficient" willingness to donate organs? Can such a thing even exist? Is not the term itself very telling? We are basically saying that the donation should by no means remain something private, absolutely voluntary, and radically removed from the will of the state but instead amounts to a moral obligation. Moreover, we refer to an organ "donation" and by using this term we essentially express the idea that the donation can be nothing other than a gift. Every donation, according to the meaning of the term, should be a gift. Even from a legal standpoint, the donation is regarded as a gift. Yet how can a donation be a gift when we refer to a "demand" for organs? Can there be a demand for gifts? Is this not a contradiction in terms?

Donation Must Not Become a Civic Duty

The entire nature of the debate reveals that the political system and the health care system have essentially rescinded the gift character of the donation and seek to implicitly elevate it to almost a civic duty. The term donation essentially implies that this donation is a unique event, an exception, at least something special. When we now seek to turn the uniqueness of the generous donation into a general rule, a matter of course and normality, then we leave the realm of the donation and enter a very different realm, namely that of the civic duty.

Transplantation medicine is squandering its potential by launching moral appeals and inoculating citizens with a guilty conscience without discussing deep-seated fears openly and honestly with the public. Transplantation medicine pursues noble goals and does valuable work. It really has nothing to hide! Therefore, it should discuss all the doubts of the nonmedical public completely openly. The vast majority of these doubts can be quickly eliminated. Think, for example, of the widespread fear that as a potential organ donor one could be excluded from therapeutic options too early. Such doubts can easily be addressed because they are unfounded. Yet it would be putting trust at risk if one were to begin dismissing all the public's doubts as irrational. Many doubts must be taken seriously and may not be trivialized or swept off the table with a single sentence. On the contrary, they must be examined more closely. And by these doubts I mean all doubts that pertain to the people directly affected, the donors themselves.

The perspective of the recipient has always dominated in the debates about organ donation. This is because people have mistakenly proceeded from the assumption that moralizing the donation is necessary to encourage willingness to donate. The media have taken this up because it is possible to produce a great emotional impact in that manner. Yet this has led to a situation where the perspective of the donor is neglected far too often. This is an ominous development because potential donors ask exactly those questions that have to do with themselves and their fate, such as: How will I feel? What will be done with me? How do family members feel? Transplantation medicine has not addressed these questions sufficiently, although there is no reason to keep anything secret. On the contrary, its task is to speak openly about what donating an organ really means. It means that the donor must forgo a peaceful conclusion to the process of dying. He must forgo giving his family members an opportunity to take their leave in an atmosphere of tranquility. He must ultimately be connected to machines, placed on a respirator, and not left in peace. He must tolerate being regarded at the end of life as a source of usable organs and not as an immutable individual. He must receive medications at the end of life not because it is good for him but because they are necessary to allow his organs to be used. Donating an organ involves a renunciation; it involves a sacrifice. These sacrifices are rarely mentioned because it is feared that speaking openly about these truths would decrease people's willingness to donate. Yet in doing so the medical profession underestimates the altruistic attitude of many people who would be willing to make this sacrifice for a good purpose but who want to be taken seriously and be honestly informed about the actual sacrifices instead of being pacified.

Is Brain Death the Death of the Person?

The medical profession must also speak openly about something else, namely brain death. Many people who are convinced of the merits of donating organs assume that they would be "dead anyway" when the organs are removed. They assume that they will be available as corpses, but they lack an adequate understanding of the status of a brain dead person. Many people who decide to donate organs do not exactly know what brain death means. They do not understand that brain dead people do not appear any different from other patients on a respirator who could soon regain their health and no longer need it. Many people do not realize that brain dead patients look alive because no one talks openly about brain death. Yet we must talk about it.

If transplantation medicine does not assume the duty of providing this information itself, then this will really create a situation of uncertainty and confusion in which many rumors will circulate. Yet these discussions must be conducted with a sense of proportion. It does not help to merely say that brain death is simply the death of the person. This is how the law has defined it and it is therefore formally correct, but in real life, it still represents a challenge for those involved. The medical profession must voluntarily inform people that although brain dead patients are dead by definition and have entered an irreversible process, they will not be perceived as dead people in real-life situations. The medical descriptions and definitions are far removed from what people actually perceive. Therefore, the medical profession itself must help people cope with this disparity between the scientific definition and what they perceive in a real-life situation. This is possible as long as it is made clear that this process is irreversible. But we must speak about the difference between a brain dead person and a corpse. And we must make it clear that we feel responsible even and especially for the brain dead person, that we show him respect, and will never turn him into an object that we can use as we see fit.

The Definition of Brain Death

Significantly, the debate about brain death and its definition was not initially conducted in the context of organ transplantation. It was first mentioned when the first artificial respirators were introduced in the 1950s and the question repeatedly arose as to how long artificial respiration should be continued or, respectively, at what point it could be discontinued. In this context, it occurred to people to say that respiration was recommended as long as the brain remained functional. When a commission at Harvard Medical School defined brain death as the death of the person in 1968, these deliberations occurred primarily in the context of passive euthanasia. As a result, it is historically incorrect to say that brain death was only invented to facilitate transplantation. Surgeons made use of this definition nonetheless, and soon brain death became a criterion for the removal of one or more organs in transplantation medicine as well. Since 1968, it has been regarded as a proven fact that brain death is the death of the person. The commission emphasized that as soon as the brain ceased to function, one could assume that not only process of dying was irreversible but also and most importantly the collapse of the entire body was occurring. This commission's assertion was that the brain is the central organ that acts as an integrator for the entire body. The death of the brain is therefore the dissolution of the complete whole, the end of the organism in the sense of a functional whole.[42]

Until then, it had not been necessary to give any thought to the exact time and course of this collapse because people were allowed to die when irreversible cardiac arrest occurred. When death is allowed, several processes occur concurrently: The heart stops, the brain (the most sensitive organ) dies within a few minutes, and the disintegration of the entire body begins. These processes form what may be considered a whole. The development of resuscitation methods and artificial respiration resulted in the separation of these processes. In intensive care units, not only are these processes decoupled from each other, but their order is reversed as well. Whereas in natural death circulatory collapse occurs first and then the brain dies, it is now the case that after resuscitation the circulatory system remains functional but the brain may already have "died." The Harvard commission of 1968 made it clear that even where the circulatory system remains functional, the brain may have stopped working. And because the commission maintained the brain was the integrator, the hub of all processes, one could no longer speak of a living body despite the still functional circulatory function. Many supporters of the brain death definition see the body of a brain dead person as nothing more than a conglomerate of perfused organs that are no longer interconnected to form a living organism. Yet it is precisely this point that has repeatedly come under heavy attack in recent years.

In the meantime, it has been demonstrated that brain dead people maintained on respirators exhibit numerous bodily functions that indicate that they are still integrated into a whole body. For example, brain dead patients have been observed to develop fevers and exhibit immune defenses. Sexual maturation and growth have been observed in brain dead children. Brain dead patients have been seen to respond to certain stimuli with an increased pulse and elevated blood pressure and even with the excretion of stress hormones. Finally, pregnant brain dead women have been able to maintain their pregnancy for months and give birth to healthy children.[43] Moreover, new imaging modalities have been able to demonstrate electrical brain activity

113

in over 10% of brain dead patients.[44] Therefore, scientists have recommended that mandatory diagnostic imaging studies be prescribed to supplement the previous practice of diagnosing brain death primarily on the basis of clinical evidence.[45] Imaging modalities such as functional magnetic resonance imaging (fMRI) and positron emission tomography (PET) can detect brain activity significantly more precisely and reliably.

What is the significance of these new findings? They illustrate that diagnosing brain death involves two different problems. The first problem is straightforward and relates to the reliability of the diagnostic methods. It is self-evident that improved technology allows more reliable diagnostics. And for that reason the current exploration of optimized diagnostic methods in the interest of avoiding misdiagnoses is a perfectly normal process. The misdiagnoses do not call brain death diagnostics as such into question, but only how it is performed. The second question that these findings pose is far more complex and far-reaching. It is this: Can brain death really be equated to the death of the person? The Harvard commission's hypothesis was that equating the two was permissible because the brain had an integrative function for the body as a whole. These new findings disprove precisely this hypothesis. They illustrate that whereas the brain is an important organ, possibly the most important organ of all for maintaining human biological life, many complex functions of human life can be maintained even without an intact brain. The brain is thus not the body's only coordination center. On the contrary, the body can also maintain itself by means of integrating functions that lie outside the brain. Thus, it is the entire body that maintains life, not the brain alone. There is a lot to suggest that the body's central power of integration cannot be localized in any one part of the body but remains a power of the body as a whole.

On the Limits of Scientific Explanations

The virulent question that arises in conjunction with brain death is this: Why can we observe functions in a brain dead patient that we would never find in a corpse? Many physicians now maintain that these observable functions are an illusion because they only simulate life where we could not actually speak of a living body. They maintain nothing less than that all the functions described are merely the mechanical result of the artificial maintenance of respiration and circulation. However, it is difficult to imagine such a clear-cut causal relationship between artificial respiration and the fact that pregnant brain dead women can maintain the pregnancy for months and then give birth to healthy children. Do these functions only simulate the living state or are they an expression of that which is living?

In the "brain death debate," it is ultimately a matter of how we should interpret the phenomena of "vitality" described earlier. Whereas some interpret them as an expression of a power of integration and thus as a sign of the continued presence of a living organism, others interpret the same phenomena as a less complex power that does not allow us to infer total integration. Here it is obviously a matter of the uncertainties in interpreting the phenomena described. We must recognize that these uncertainties are precisely that—uncertainties— and we must understand that we are not talking about facts but ultimately about an unavoidable social process of forging a consensus with respect to the question of how much integration must be present for us to speak of a living person. These questions are not only academic in nature; rather, they reflect the daily routine in transplantation medicine.

Many people who deal with brain dead patients have difficulty with the fact that these patients cannot be perceived as dead. This applies to family members who have to take their leave from a person who looks alive and has "only" been defined as dead. But this also applies to the nursing staff. Many nurses feel this definition contradicts their own immediate experience when they care for brain dead patients. In caring for brain dead patients, they become aware of the discrepancy between the definition and the actual action because they want to care for living people, not dead people. The status of the brain dead person is difficult to determine. It is hard to recognize him as dead because the body does not appear like a dead body. Yet the body hosts the human identity and this makes it difficult for nursing staff and family members to cope with equating brain death to death without qualms.

It would be devastating for transplantation medicine if the suspicion that the definition of the time of death has essentially been adapted to the practical necessities of organ transplantation were to be left unchallenged. That would weaken the basic trust in all of medicine. To this extent, the appropriate gesture on the part of the medical profession cannot be that of indicating certainty and clear determinability. Physicians would be well advised to spell out the uncertainties here and even to accept what may be irresolvable ignorance rather than suggesting a clarity which in the definition of death—as a phenomenon of the entire human being and his culture—can never really exist.

An Approach to Humane Transplant Medicine

In my opinion, it is therefore crucial to a relationship of trust that the physicians involved in the consultations and the operation always appear as physicians—and to be a physician means to pursue a helping profession. Even the transplantation specialist wants to help above all.

But this help is often understood too narrowly. It should not apply only to the recipient but equally to the donor and especially his family members. That is a very important point! Because this seems to me to be another reason for this subtle mistrust. Many people who are relatives of organ donors report how little anybody looked after them once they had given their consent. And these relatives are the ones who then have unpleasant memories of organ removal and transplantation medicine. I think it is not necessarily inherent in the matter itself that relatives feel this way. On the contrary, how they are treated is important, to what extent they are seen as the addressees of the treatment team.

Mourning and Parting

Family members have existential needs and concerns that appear to stand in the way of the smooth "flow" of an efficient organ removal procedure. Yet it would be best to take these needs seriously. The physicians must not appear to be "organ trustees." They must also be attendants to family members who have a need to take leave of their father, their friend, their daughter, their wife, or sister. These people are close to the brain dead person even when he is brain dead and has become an organ donor. In my opinion, it is essential to treat these needs with absolute respect. For it is difficult to take leave of a person when his body does not show manifestly obvious signs of his death. Therefore, it is important for people to be prepared for this discrepancy between the appearance and the declaration of death by definition. Only then can they take leave of their family member even though they may still perceive him as alive. If people are subjected to this situation unprepared, they will have traumatic memories of it and it will leave behind emotions that are hardly conducive to the relationship of trust between the individual and medicine as a whole. Therefore, these challenges should be met head on. Family members

117

should be prepared, and they should be supported in the situation itself with a maximum of empathy.

One other consideration is very important for the family members: they must be able to mourn. And it is important for transplantation specialists that they also feel responsible for supporting family members in their process of grieving. I ask myself whether establishing structures for aftercare might not be an eminently commendable confidence-building measure. For example, it should be possible to conduct a discussion with family members a few weeks after the organ donation to give them the opportunity to "unload" all the pent-up questions that have been troubling them in the meantime. Such a discussion should be scheduled right away when they take their leave of the donor. I feel such aftercare is crucial because only in this manner will we convey to family members that feeling that they are being taken seriously. We will convey the feeling that the donor is not merely an organ supplier and they themselves are not merely signatures on a consent form, rather that the hospital continues to feel responsible for the donor and his family and continues to offer support.

Responsibility for the Organ Donor

Trustworthy and responsible transplantation medicine means more than merely offering recipients a suitable organ. In my opinion, medical care for the recipient should be seen in a larger context. For the recipients in particular, it is important to know that that they have received an organ that they were entitled to because they were the next on the list and not because they have won some sort of shady lottery where resources are traded under the counter. Another tragic aspect of the fraud scandals is that the recipients have been unsettled in this manner. I am convinced they need more than that. To be able to live well with the organ, they are utterly dependent on the feeling that the organ was bestowed upon them with deep conviction from the bottom of the heart. We owe it not only to the donors but also to the recipients that they receive an organ that has been given absolutely voluntarily on the basis of a deep conviction and in full awareness of all the implications, not by someone who was trapped. Therefore, it is in the interest of the recipients in particular that we do not tolerate any half-hearted decisions with respect to organ donation. The trustworthiness of transplantation medicine hinges on realizing that a no from the family members is still better than a half-hearted yes. And that a yes to organ donation is really a blessing only when it is the expression of a process of maturation. For this reason, we should welcome the German "Law Regulating the Decision Solution in the Transplantation Law" that came into effect in 2012 and provides for "regularly putting" every citizen above the age of 16 "in the position of seriously considering his own willingness to donate" so that everyone can go through this process of maturation. No one has to make decision here and now and definitely not a final one. The media in particular must simply recognize that for many people it is asking too much to make a considered decision on the spot. There should be an atmosphere in which this inability is clearly accepted as an understandable condition and there is no coercion.

The German Federal Central Office for Health Education (BZgA) informs the public about the most important questions regarding every aspect of organ and tissue donation in an effort to support individual decision making. It answers questions such as:
- *What does the implementation of the decision solution mean for citizens?*
- *Will my decision be registered by the health insurance funds?*
- *How is organ and tissue donation regulated in Germany?*
- *What requirements must be met for organ and tissue donation?*

- *What is an organ donor ID?*
- *Can you change your decision about organ and tissue donation?*

(Source: www.organspende-info.de)

Every Decision to Donate an Organ Is of Vital Importance, Even for the Donor

Now everything depends on how well the public is informed and how hospitals deal with the proxy consent of family members. In the interest of trustworthy medicine, I feel it is imperative to plan the informative discussions in such a way as to exclude any risk that the family members might later regret their decision. Before we accept regret, it would be better not to demand a decision of them. The new law in particular will give rise a culture in which the transplantation representatives, who under Section 9b (2) of the transplantation law are charged with providing appropriate support for the donors' family members, will assume a very special responsibility.

The representatives' goal should be to regard themselves as unbiased attendants of a good decision who give the family members the feeling of being able to decide without any pressure. In this context, I feel it is absolutely unacceptable to convey, even indirectly, the impression that consent is morally superior than rejection. Precisely such a suggestive approach to the family members would create mistrust because then the family members would no longer have the feeling that the medical profession gives consideration to the donor as well as the recipient. Therefore, it is important even in light of transplantation medicine's noble goals that we respect the fact that every decision for or against organ donation is a very important decision for the donor, one whose significance to him can hardly be overestimated.

The decision to donate an organ is a vital matter for the donor as well! Therefore, it must always be regarded as a highly personal matter that must not be motivated by advertising campaigns.

Advertising seems to me to be a great obstacle to the relationship of trust because it has a suggestive character. It pursues a certain purpose and as a result is fundamentally manipulative. In other words, the aspect of persuasion is an integral part of advertising; otherwise, it would not be advertising at all. Because of this, advertising misses the mark in a very special way when it comes to the matter of trust. Transplantation medicine simply has no need of advertising for itself because its high moral goal is obvious. I find all these beautiful pictures, these hidden appeals to compassion irritating only because they kindle the public's suspicion that the advertising is being used to conceal something less moral. And yet the problem of advertising is not that it might be misrepresenting something. The problem lies more in the selective choice of what is true. That means that advertising always involves a reduction in complexity: it makes reality simpler than it is. It suggests that deciding to donate an organ is trivial and perfectly normal. And it is precisely this suggestion that contradicts common sense and ultimately scares people off. Therefore, people must again be made aware that transplantation medicine is valuable in itself and never deserved to be wrapped in advertising slogans.

It would be important for every one of us to get the feeling that transplantation medicine is not primarily about receiving as many organs as possible but about helping people to reach a decision that makes sense to them by giving comprehensive unfiltered information. Only then can the organs donated on the basis of conviction be implanted to the benefit of many severely ill people. Maybe we could say that the

121

trust in transplantation medicine will be fully restored when everybody involved actually witnesses on a daily basis a vibrant culture of dealing humanely with the sick and the dying as well as with brain dead people and corpses. This behavior, which must be respectful and pious, ultimately determines how transplantation medicine will be viewed. Thus, we can help people not only by increasing the transplantation rates but also by means of a daily culture of deep respect. Trust will consolidate precisely when as many people as possible begin to feel this deep respect and realize that this practiced compassion is extended to the recipients just as it is to the donors and their family members. Unfortunately, until now it has been the case in everyday clinical practice that a lot of effort is invested in discussions with the family members of the donors until they give their consent, after which the contact abruptly breaks off.

Transplant Medicine Is Relationship-Centered Medicine

There are many people for whom the simple knowledge that they can make their own organs available to someone else is very fulfilling. Many people even speak of fulfilling a purpose in this context. The thought of helping other people even beyond their own death has something sustaining for them. And according to everything I have experienced, the recipients experience it the same way. They feel a deep gratitude to the donor. They invariably relate to him. We must think of these people when we ask what sort of culture should characterize transplantation medicine and how trust can be established. These people illustrate that transplantation medicine is not merely a matter of a technological process but of nothing less than human relationships. It is about people who enter a relationship with each other although they have never met. One anticipated the relationship as he was still healthy, the other experiences it physically.

As paradoxical as it may sound, donating an organ occurs within a relationship even when the donor is a brain dead person.

Transplantation medicine is not merely the practiced application of a technique; rather, it is medicine that involves relationships. And our trust will strengthen transplantation medicine when it reveals itself in its everyday practice as medicine that involves relationships. Of course, there are very good reasons why the donor and the recipient remain anonymous and the system does not permit a relationship between them, with the exception of live donations in which relatives or partners donate organs. Yet the person who feels sustained by the knowledge that he will give his organs to others can do so because he enters into an anticipated relationship. The donation links his life and fate in a certain way to the life and fate of another human being. Maybe this is what is fascinating about transplantation medicine, that two people are brought together in a certain sense by the physician's skill. If we view transplantation medicine from this perspective, then it becomes clear that we do not need an advertising campaign but need to reflect on that fact that it is nothing less than this: relationship-centered medicine.

Chapter 6
On the Value of Age, Beyond the Fitness Imperative

We are living in an age of paradoxes. People are living ever longer but nobody wants to be old. If we have to be old, then we should at least be old youthfully. Nowhere is this mindset more apparent than in the current boom in anti-aging medicine. But is good old age only fit old age? What is the meaning of being old? Is there a meaning to it at all? This chapter examines the history of thought and other conceptions of old age, and shows how it is a phase of life in which one is endowed with a particular sagacity, with a resolving and deepening appreciation for the essential conditions of human existence.

Recently, I came across an advertising slogan for an anti-aging skin cream: "Getting older? No problem. Slowing down is out of the question for me!" This advertising slogan clearly illustrates the attitude toward aging that many parts of today's society live with. According to them, being old is only good if one "does not slow down." The implicit message of this advertising is that the only person who ages well is the one who does not allow the signature features of being old, among them slowing down. Moreover, if one begins to slow down in old age, then it is one's own fault; it is the result of one's own omissions. Thus, we are well advised to address old age early—so as to avoid old age itself. This is the paradoxical message that this advertising ultimately conveys and, at the same time, it is the wish of large parts of society. Old age should not be overcome, mastered, or fulfilled but preferably done away with entirely because ultimately it reminds us of transience and is seen as a harbinger of our unavoidable death.

"So That the Arc of Life May Be Complete ..."

The more the central theme of youthfulness is valued—and that is the fundamental intention of anti-aging medicine—the more old age appears and is thought of only as something deficient. It is then only the "no longer," and the more it appears as such a "no longer," the more we lose sight of the deep truth that life without old age can no longer be complete. We forget that all of life consists of cycles. What is special about old age can only be understood in light of this cyclical pattern, that means in relation to the other phases of life. Especially in ancient times, it was thought that each period of life had its own special characteristic and particular significance. All of life's seasons should be recognized as valuable in their intrinsic meaning, and one could understand all of life as a process of change "from the active life to the contemplative life."[46] On the other hand, we tend to declare the active middle phase of life as the model for the whole of life.

I do not intend in any way to belittle the tribulations that arise when one can do progressively less, quite the opposite! These tribulations cannot be denied and, as was known even in ancient times, they are at times difficult to bear. Aging is to a certain extent invariably associated with a certain suffering, with suffering that manifests itself in the body but also a suffering from that which is past and irretrievably gone, suffering from a life that knows an irredeemable past and only a very limited future. But does that which anti-aging medicine provides actually alleviate this suffering of old age? It seems to me that the more medicine regards age as an enemy it must fight, the more difficult it becomes to age. For anti-aging suggests this: if I only make

125

an effort and do a lot (or buy a lot) for it, then I can avoid slowing down. It encourages clinging to the attitude that only one phase of life, namely the middle one, is valuable and even justified. It entrenches the dependence on the products of the health industry and blinds people to the insight that slowing down in old age is part of a complete life. The philosopher and theologian Romano Guardini (1885–1968) put it in a nutshell:

> "The ancients spoke of the 'ars moriendi,' of the art of dying, by which they meant that there is wrong dying and right dying: simply running out and perishing, but also becoming finished and complete, the final realization of the form of being. If that applies to death, then all the more to aging."[47]

Guardini challenges us to expressly include aging in the image that we make of our existence ("so that the arc of life may be complete") and not simply as a waste product of the "real" life, namely the active life. The philosopher Thomas Rentsch goes in a similar direction, albeit an anti-theological one, when he refers to aging as "life's becoming definitive" and sees in it a chance "of becoming oneself."[48]

A person's becoming human, his maturing, indeed his fulfillment ultimately include recognizing that all of life is part of this process of aging. The more anti-aging medicine propagates the ideal of an ageless life, the more it leads people astray and undercuts people's fundamental capacity for approaching old age not only defensively but also in a fundamental attitude of acceptance—also as an acceptance of themselves.

Anti-Aging Is Suppression of the Knowledge of One's Own Finiteness

The problem of anti-aging thus lies in the attitude of "good aging" which stands thinly veiled behind the products being extolled. Anti-aging suggests—as our slogan at the beginning well demonstrates—that good aging can only be aging that continues to wrap itself in the cloak of youth. Improving an aging face, having wrinkles removed—all this is basically a desperate attempt to stop time, to erase the traces of the passage of time and all this under the delusional assumption that by erasing the traces of the passage of time one could bring back time itself. All these aspirations of hiding signs of old age converge in modern medicine. They are ultimately nothing other than an effort to dull our consciousness of our mortality, of the transience of being. We can hardly bear to be reminded of this. And thus we face the traces of time that drained from our life using a narcotic to help us forget the pain. Yet every thinking person knows that even the best narcotic is only effective for a limited time and that anesthetizing the "pain of time trickling away"[49] cannot be cure trickling time itself. For time advances inexorably and catches up with everyone. Moreover, people assume they would gain something if they could only suspend time. But exactly the opposite is true: depth and mortality—they are mutually dependent! One cannot simply want to lead an ageless life and expect that all emotional qualities will remain. That is a big mistake because the quality of feeling is linked to the awareness that our life is limited. Were we to remove the limits from life, then every feeling would necessarily change.[50]

Anti-Aging Reduces a Person to His Need to Perform

At the same time, the anti-aging aspirations also express a certain obligation to be fit and imply that age in itself loses any value as soon as it can no longer be lived in fitness. I find this message highly problematic as it is so hostile to the elderly. For it forces many elderly people with illnesses, impairments, and disabilities into isolation or even despair for the very reason that according to this message they have essentially squandered every possibility to lead a good life. This mindset regards the value of being old under the paradigm of a need to perform: dignified aging is equated to able-bodied aging. This reduces a person to his functionality, to what he can do. But does not being a human being mean more than being able-bodied? Moreover, in this perspective the good is seen in being able to do everything. The more a person can do, the more dignified his life is. But what has happened to the insight that dignified aging can be characterized by constructively dealing with the fact that an older person simply cannot do as much as a younger person? Maturity in age could precisely mean coming to terms with the experience of not being able to do everything in such a way that one gains the ability to acquire a taste for this "no longer" and precisely in doing so becomes able to achieve something like maturity and depth. Maturity and depth by accepting the limit that applies to *every* human being!

As I see it, the problems of the anti-aging trend lie in the fact that glorifying youth undermines the sensibility of the young for the value of being old. That begins with the approach of wanting to give aging people a youthful appearance using a variety of methods. Is the implied premise of equating youthfulness with beauty really so self-evident? Or is this limited perspective not in fact an expression of a limited mindset that increasingly keeps us from approaching old age confidently and serenely? With an attitude of acceptance, one would inevitably be open for the insight that not only youth but also every age can be labeled with the attribute of beauty. Yet the beauty of old age will only reveal itself to whomever who does not reject old age but initially accepts it as a part of himself, allows it to act on himself, and develops his own potential. This potential has less to do with the common qualifications of a performance society geared to youthfulness than with the ones that are intrinsic to each phase of life in its own way and which fundamentally have to do with being and existence. We tend to see old age only from the perspective of the "growing shadow of the fading light."[51] Limiting our view to the shadow in this manner is tantamount to blindness because in this way we become blind to the light that continues to shine in its own way.

Age Is a Clear View of Reality

Since ancient times, it has been regarded as a particular advantage of old age that in this phase of life man is less driven by his desires and passions, thus allowing him a clearer view of reality. Old age is often said to have an affinity to the intellectual, even the spiritual, to what Romano Guardini has referred to as a "becoming transparent for its sense." Because he is less active and instead becomes increasingly aware of the conditionality of all being and all ability, the elderly person has the opportunity to differentiate what is important from what is unimportant and what is genuinely crucial from what is thought to be crucial. To this extent, I would regard old age as a phase in which one is capable of particular insights precisely because in a certain sense one has become "impervious to bribery." One no longer has to conform to the dominant mindset because one has nothing more to lose. And one no longer has to deceive oneself because one no longer needs the illusions:

"He who wants nothing more, acquires—in compensation—the ability to see a lot." (Odo Marquard)[52]

Thus, in a certain sense it is precisely the lack of a future that prevents us in old age from being blinded by our desires and longings. Precisely because the elderly person does not have to conform to a future that he no longer has, he acquires the opportunity to see things as they are and in so doing become "capable of theory," because theory, according to the philosopher Odo Marquard born in 1928, is "what one does when there is nothing more to be done."[53] One acquires insights when the focus is no longer on actively doing, on industriousness, but on being in itself. What many people today would like to dull with the narcotic of anti-aging—the fact of having progressively less future available—represents the essential condition for a particular sagacity of old age.

Deepening the Essential Conditions of Human Existence

Not only can we ascribe a clear view of things to old age, but also we can even characterize it as radicalizing the essential conditions of human existence and allowing people significant insights—for example, the insight of being fundamentally vulnerable, defenseless, and threatened by suffering. In a certain sense, we are also rendered capable of realizing the fundamentally limited opportunities that human life affords us and thus arriving at what the ancients referred to as the wisdom of old age.[54] Even what many people see as painful, namely coming to appreciate their own finiteness, in this way becomes something positive in that a person acquires insights that tend to remain out of reach at a young age. It is through this realization and in the awareness of the finality with which life definitively concludes in old age that a person receives, according to Thomas Rentsch, the chance to "permanently distinguish what is humanly important from the many unimportant things in clarifying retrospection."[55]

Age Is a Learning Model for Society

The theologian Hans-Martin Rieger goes one step further. Particularly in light of his radicalization of the essential conditions of human existence, he sees in old age a necessary "signal function for the whole of society which for its part is tempted to exile dependency to the reservation of the fourth age."[56] Accordingly, old age is not only a key phase of life for the people in question but for the whole of society because in their confrontation with becoming old they remind us that it is not independence but dependence that represents a basic hallmark of the human being, one which he as a human being cannot shuffle off. Thus, old age can be regarded as a reminder of what defines a human being, as a reminder that man needs to avoid succumbing to the illusion of absolute feasibility. As a phase of life in which we learn and must learn to deal with limitations and losses, old age could be a continuous "patient history" for a society, helping it to remain aware of the alternating dependence relationships. Being old would then be something like a reminder of limitation and thus a "learning model for society."[57]

Precisely this aspect illustrates what a narrow perspective those people have who regard old age only as a phase of life for which society must do something. Conversely, with respect to the model character of old age, we could also say that old age does not only need something but also gives something, namely valuable insights into a depth that tend to remain out of reach for the other phases of life. Thus, one could ultimately regard old age as an educational task, as a phase of life in which "dealing constructively with one's own limits"[58] is shown and lived.

The Relationship of Dependency

Doing justice to the elderly person can only mean perceiving him in his specific quality of being old and to value him for this, and not for what he can do but for what he is: a person dependent on the support of other people. We tend today toward a narrowed understanding of dependence. That is a key problem and it is also the problem of many elderly people who cannot cope with being dependent on other people for help. Modern man sees himself as a fundamentally autonomous being and has a fraught relationship to the undeniable fact that sooner or later every person will need the help of other people to survive. In this perspective, dependence on others is seen only as destruction of autonomy. It is interpreted as the end of one's own self and as something that one can only accept with horror. This ignores the fact that the dependence on others is a basic hallmark of life, and it is entirely forgotten that dependence is not the end of autonomy but an essential condition of existing in general and thus a prerequisite for autonomy. Therefore, it is no wonder at all that people today think about dependence so shortsightedly, especially in an age in which we are beginning to weed out human life even before birth for the simple reason that it does not meet our expectations (see Chapter 2). Elderly people's self-image does not remain unscathed when they see themselves confronted with developments in which human life at its beginning can be seen as an unreasonable demand, for example, because it comes into the world with a disability. The same applies when elderly people discover that the public generally finds it good that human life with disabilities is regarded as such a great obstacle that the state even allows the killing of this life and calls this killing an act of help. More and more, the elderly person (who we already are or will inevitably be in the future) is burdened with the fear that he himself may be experienced in our society as an unreasonable demand as soon as he develops disabilities.

It is hardly noticed that such a fear of being dependent on others is tantamount to a fundamental attitude that negates life, to rendering the middle phase of life absolute, and to a narrowed understanding of being in need of help. One can be in need of help while still retaining a modicum of individual control over one's life even if this lies in the smallest acts of daily life, in the choice of one word, gesture, or expression and not another. I feel it is particularly important to foster an awareness of this potential when caring for the elderly. Comprehensively doing justice to the elderly requires an interest in how the elderly person, despite and because of being in need of help, can continue to express his distinctive personality and how he can be assisted in doing this. Therefore, it must be a central goal of society to open up new creative spaces and seek structural conditions that permit elderly people to live a life that corresponds to their own individual personality as much as possible. This means creating spaces that allow elderly people to contribute their own specific competence as elderly people, their competence as unique people—even if it is the competence to recount something or convey something by gestures, expressions, or sentence fragments.

The greatest danger lies in what one could refer to as self-stereotyping, that means applying someone else's negative attitude to one's own self, in this case accepting a self-image in which one is often regarded as a poor excuse for humanity. This attitude must be confronted! In the interest of all elderly people as in our own interest, we must learn that being old is a valuable form of the human condition, an expression of dependence that not only is to be tolerated but also has an important function for all people.

We are largely accustomed to seeing a person's autonomy as the highest purpose solely in his living entirely from and by himself, not being dependent on the conditions of his physical body and not being dependent on his fellow human beings. Such an understanding of autonomy fails to recognize the finite nature of all life. It fails to recognize that we have always lived in a relationship of dependence, not only in old age. This relationship is what makes human life possible in the first place! Whereas it is expressed more strongly in childhood and old age, dependence as such is not specific to or a peculiarity of old age but is a fundamental structure of our entire life.

> We must again develop a feeling for the fact that even in its phases of best performance life is invariably also a life in a relationship of dependence.

We can do nothing by ourselves. We are dependent throughout life, dependent on relationships to other people and thus dependent on the care, recognition, cooperation, and help of other people. And this is where old age acquires a special meaning. For old age reminds us of this. In it, dependence occurs in a radicalized form. It is also a reminder of what the human being is: a finite being that cannot exist alone.

The Old Person Gives Us Something

Yet old age teaches us more than that. It teaches us that we can master life not only by being active. It teaches us that a person can respond to decreasing physical performance not only with more training and more activity but also, as many elderly people show us, by rethinking and realigning his goals in life.[59] Seeing an elderly person and his way of life makes it clear to all of us that preferences and life goals are relative. We can anticipate that very different values will become important later. Old age, so I am convinced, makes us receptive to the fact that what appears so important today can be of little value tomorrow. Ultimately, old age gives us cause to reflect on the fact that satisfaction with life can depend on goals beyond those we can even imagine in our high-performance middle years.

> Old age can be a sort of magnifying glass that focuses on what is important in life.

The elderly person has different ways of shaping his life than the person who is "in the middle of life." This is obvious from the ability to find joy in the little things of everyday life and to rediscover the uniqueness of what was perfectly ordinary before. The specific approach to life that many elderly people realize becomes apparent in their behavior toward relationships, for example, when they avoid superficial contacts or friendships with ulterior motives. Finally, it becomes apparent in how many people lose their fear of death and develop a new attitude toward life, death, and mortality. With this attitude, one ceases to fear one's own finiteness and undertakes a fundamental reckoning with the fact that one is limited oneself. "I enjoy living now much more than earlier; suddenly I like the daily routine which had never interested me before," announced Austrian author Gerhard Roth on the occasion of his 70th birthday. "And now I like everything without pause, the shapes of leaves, the changing seasons, meetings with people, when Sturm Graz wins a game. The sum of these things gives me more strength than before. I don't see my end approaching so threateningly. The coming and the disappearing has something to do with the whole universe, which is moving apart and will one day collapse. Everything is equipped with an end, why should it be any different with me?"[60] Naturally, it is difficult for a person with many ailments to see things this way. And yet a great potential lies in our attitude toward the ailments. It always depends on how we see life, whether we see it as a life in decline or whether we still recognize the vitality in this life, maybe even recognize it anew especially in light of the ailments.

We must establish a new culture of dealing with old age and the elderly, a culture that is not guided only by what we should do for the elderly but that remains open to the insight that it is they who can give us so much. Elderly people do not only want to have their needs taken care of; they want to be accepted as valuable people and be treated with respect and enthusiasm. The fact that many elderly people no longer find their way to these feelings is due in no small measure to the fact that care for the elderly, like care in general, is increasingly understood as "close-contact service" in which it is a matter of addressing needs and not of interpersonal contact in a meeting between two people. Elderly people do not only need a functioning system of care that has learned how to ensure personal hygiene as effectively as possible. Above all, they need genuine personalities who are interested in them and, notwithstanding all the required care, express to them that they are seen as important and uniquely interesting people. Stopwatch care that devotes more time to documenting how long it took to wash a person, where the caregiver is thinking about the next patient while washing this one, such care may be good at providing for basic needs but it has forgotten how to genuinely encounter the person. And the people thus cared for will inevitably see themselves as people who only make other people work.

Ultimately, we all feel valued when society indicates to us that what we can contribute is valuable. The elderly person who no longer stands in the midst of life's demands but has become "capable of theory"—observing, knowing, summarizing—can become engaged in volunteer activities or he can simply tell stories or simply be there, be responsive. Existence for others can be active giving but it can also be simple existence. In contrast to the person in the active middle phase of life, the elderly person gives simply by his existence, simply by being. He gives by means of the life he himself has lived, by the way in which he has lived and written his own life story. This lived life for which he has taken responsibility radiates something. The dignity of the elderly person is the result of this life alone, a dignity that, as Guardini emphasizes, comes not from performance but from being.

Being old may well ultimately make us receptive to the feeling that every person is given and that this givenness of the person can open up a valuable new fundamental attitude in light of old age. This is the fundamental attitude of deep gratitude for what is, for what seems to be the most trivial thing a person can do, what is seemingly the least important thing he encounters, what seems to be the slightest thing he is given—indeed ultimately gratitude for the fact that we exist at all. Yet we exist only at the cost of our transience. And the more transient we can experience ourselves, the more valuable the moment will be to us. Awareness of the preciousness of the moment consciously lived is not the exclusive privilege of the elderly. Yet I would like to live in a society in which we take this message all the more seriously when we know it comes from an elderly person. The elderly person has a lot to tell us. We need only be prepared to give him a voice.

Chapter 7
Living Wills - Are Forms Replacing Dialogue?

The living will is always praised as the silver bullet for meeting the challenge of dying in the modern world. It is intended to do justice to the patient's own self-determined will and to his autonomous decision to refuse medical life support should he be in a situation of radical dependence on others. Yet can autonomy be so easily called into play? Does not genuine self-determination require the relationship, the discussion, the care—especially at the end of life? Proceeding from a patient's story, this chapter will reflect upon the advantages and limits of the living will and will make an appeal for a culture of dependence and communicative coexistence.

The Living Will

Geared to efficiency and self-determination, the one-sided thinking of our age becomes particularly obvious in the way the subject of "dying" is treated in public discussions. It is not a coincidence that the reaction to the challenges of dying has been the particularly vehement political demand to enshrine the living will in a statute.

> In Germany, the living will was first regulated by statute on September 1, 2009, when the Care Act was expanded. A living will is a written statement expressing a person's desires in the event he is no longer able to express informed consent; it primarily pertains to medical measures or, respectively, the refusal of life support measures.

The living will actually offers many opportunities. I will mention these first because my intent is not to criticize the living will but to advocate its prudent use. The advantages of the living will lie in the fact that the reason for drafting one can lead to the person to reflect upon his own finiteness well in advance. The living will thus provide an opportunity to confront one's own death. And the new Care Act that gave the living will legally binding force offers the opportunity of providing greater certainty of action. The essential content can be summarized in five key points:

1. *The living will must be expressed in writing.*
2. *Notarization is not required.*
3. *The living will has no limitation in scope; it applies not only to severe illnesses but also to every condition that the signatory describes.*
4. *The guardian is crucial to the execution of the instrument; this means that the will primarily addresses the guardian so that this person will see to it that the instructions are followed.*
5. *Involving the guardianship court is only necessary when there is dissension between the guardian and the physician. In all other situations, that is, whenever the physician follows the guardian's evaluation, no court is involved.*

Item 5 in particular was not entirely clear prior to the law. Since then it has been established that no other authority is required as long as the guardian (in most cases family members) and the physician are in agreement. This last item in particular places great responsibility on the guardian's shoulders but also the physicians'. To actually exercise this responsibility properly, one must be aware of the limits of the living will. One should reflect on these limits not in an effort to contest the validity of the living will (which even from a purely legal standpoint is not possible) but to allow a more nuanced way of dealing with it.

A Patient's Story

As an introduction to critical reflection, I recount a patient's story that was cause for a clinical ethics consultation.

> *An 83-year-old woman is resuscitated by the emergency physician at home following a syncope (loss of consciousness) and is brought to the hospital's emergency room. There she is diagnosed with severe constriction of the coronary arteries, necessitating double bypass surgery. After surgery, she is admitted to the intensive care unit. The woman's circulatory system is quickly stabilized and she is taken off the respirator. The woman later regains consciousness and is transferred to the day ward with a good neurological prognosis. There she develops a severe lung infection within 4 days which necessitates transferring her back to the intensive care unit. The patient is no longer responsive but her condition is nonetheless described as stable. From a medical perspective, a good prognosis can be assumed insofar as the lung infection is treated. Yet this again requires artificial respiration. Despite her advanced age and patient history, the physicians assume that after several days on the respirator and antibiotic therapy, the patient could recover sufficiently to be released from the hospital and sent home, where she could continue to live with a good quality of life. The patient's family members note that further treatment would not be in keeping with the patient's will and therefore ask to refrain from any further artificial respiration. Years previously, the patient had signed a living will stipulating that "in case of an incurable illness [...]" she did "not desire to be kept alive by artificial means." In the living will she further stipulates that she should be allowed to die if there were no "reasonable chance" of her recovering or if she had to experience "severe suffering" and her "conscious existence" were no longer possible.*

> *The family members note that the patient had already refused a particularly oppressive medical treatment in younger years. At the time she*

had already undergone surgery for breast and bowel cancer and in both cases categorically refused chemotherapy even if this could possibly have cured her. Although she had become progressively weaker prior to being admitted to the hospital, she had not wanted to accept hospital treatment. She even explicitly refused implantation of a cardiac pacemaker earlier. Her fundamental attitude, according to the family members, consists in forgoing medical interventions to the greatest extent possible and in accepting death should it come down to that. From the perspective of the family members, further intensive care treatment would not do justice to the patient, only transferring her to a palliative ward or into a hospice.

This patient's story graphically illustrates that decision making in broad areas of medicine cannot follow purely medical considerations. Because whether or not artificial respiration is justifiable in this specific case cannot be decided simply on the basis of a description of radiographic findings and expertise in pharmacology and micro-biology, but only by applying ethical standards.

The ethical question here is whether one does justice to the patient by allowing her to die. The family members note that allowing her to die would be in keeping with the patient's will. Yet how are we supposed to deal with this appraisal? The living will can be helpful here, yet the requirement stipulated by the patient for forgoing therapy (incurable ailment that does not permit conscious existence) is not unequivocally fulfilled in the current situation. The recourse to the patient's general standards of value as described by her family members is also important. Obviously, she is critical of conventional medicine and has refused many recommended treatments in the past. Yet doubts arise as to whether this attitude of refusal can be assumed in the specific situation at hand. Thus, the treatment team notes that in the phase after the operation when the patient was responsive, their concurring

141

impression was that the patient did not indicate that she did not approve of the previous course of treatment or that she did not wish any further treatment.

The consultation between the treatment team and the family members initially failed to produce a consensus. The new Care Act provides for a decision by the guardianship court (see earlier) in such a situation of conflicting attitudes between the treatment team and the family members. However, everyone involved felt that petitioning the court would not be the best solution. As a result, a second expanded consultation took place between the family members and the treatment team including the entire management during which it arose that initial findings suggested the course of treatment would be positive. In light of this positive course, the decision was reached to initially continue treatment but avoid any escalation of the therapy.

This patient's story illustrates that the living will alone was not able to provide absolute certainty in this case. Rather, it was only the living will in the context of the patient's prior history and also in the context of her current behavior that led to a decision. We need to examine the living will more closely particularly with respect to its limits.

Autonomy and Care

The living will has repeatedly been praised in political debates as an instrument for safeguarding the patient's autonomy.[61] Respecting the patient's autonomy is a fundamental precept of every treatment because it means nothing other than respecting the person in his uniqueness, singularity, and fundamental immutability. Failing to respect autonomy would violate the person's dignity. Therefore, respecting patient autonomy is not an obligation that the new law has recently introduced; rather, it is a fundamental precept of every treatment if we want to speak of respectful behavior. Thus, the discussion about the living will has not posed the question—long resolved—of whether or not autonomy should be respected. On the contrary, it gives rise to the question of whether the living will has actually done what it was promised to do in the debates, namely strengthen autonomy. Here uncertainty remains.

Autonomy Is Often Possible Only through Care

Here we should first consider that autonomy in the context of sickness is not simply something that one can conserve and then activate as if by a mouse click. Autonomy is something that must first be developed anew in light of the crisis situation. The patient must first relate to his sickness in order to be in any position to deal with the end of his life in a self-determined manner. This relating requires time, effort, consultations, and advice. As there is no provision for any of this in the law, it is completely ignored. Of course, it is possible for a person to draft a living will that precisely expresses what constitutes his individuality. Yet it will often be the case that people will first have to find their way to their attitude by exchanging information, asking questions, and gaining experience. The law, which does not require any education of the patient and also does not specify any other criteria by which to evaluate how well informed a patient is, certainly strengthens the self-confident and knowledgeable person who is experienced with disease. Whether it also strengthens patients who have had little experience, exposure, and exchange of information and are less self-confident is open to question. In any case, there will always be many people whose autonomy will only really be respected when someone is there to help them arrive at a well-considered and mature decision about themselves.

Will My Attitude Be the Same Tomorrow as It Is Today?

The second uncertainty lies in the possible discrepancy that can arise between today's attitude and tomorrow's, which must necessarily remain a hypothetical prediction. It is, of course, true of many other situations that we must often assume responsibility for decisions that may only become relevant later. With respect to dying as an exceptional situation for the human being, this weighs more heavily insofar as when people are healthy they tend (as many studies here have shown) to imagine their own attitude to an illness too negatively.[62] Here, too, it would be very important for physicians in particular to make an effort to inform patients. Yet there is no such requirement anywhere. I feel that we can only ensure that living wills will be dealt with properly if we always bear this fundamental fallibility in mind and avoid a false sense of security that could ultimately prove illusory.

> The great danger of the statutory provisions lies precisely in the false security that codified law suggests to many people.

Uncertainties in Interpretation

The third uncertainty lies in language. Proponents of the statutory solution all too often proceed from the assumption that words are able to precisely express exactly what is to be done later. Precisely, this assumption represents a fundamental misunderstanding. For a written document to be understood as a guideline for action, it must first be interpreted. One need not be a structuralist to recognize that this can be a very complex and extremely demanding process. This applies especially to terms that in themselves are rather unspecific, such as "inhumane death" or "life support." These generic terms can include a wide variety of specific things. What exactly does a patient mean by "inhumane death"? What measures fall under "life support"—artificial respiration or, for example, the administration of antibiotics? Yet even when the terms are more precise and more specific, one will still have to interpret. Being able to interpret well usually requires one to become familiar with the patient's environment because this will provide information about how this or that expression the patient used is best understood. Taking the document by itself and attempting to derive a guideline for action from it without becoming familiar with the patient and his environment is not the proper way to deal with a living will.

Forms Cannot Substitute Relationships

Living wills can really represent a strengthening of autonomy only if the will is not regarded as a replacement for a relationship. This relationship is also possible and especially necessary with a patient who is unable or no longer able to express informed consent, for example, a patient with dementia or a mental disability. Especially in dealing with these "weak" patients, one will only achieve good medical care by engaging with the patient, becoming involved with him, and attempting to listen to him even if he is unable to express informed consent. The living will has not made becoming involved with patients obsolete and dispensable, quite the opposite! Living wills must be followed unconditionally (provided certain criteria are met), but following them only does justice to the patient when a relationship has first been established and following the will is not regarded as a substitute for such a relationship.

This is not merely an academic issue because many physicians felt relieved when the new law on living wills came into effect. They felt this way because they hope to be relieved of their responsibility.

A relief for the physicians because they think that where there is a written will they will no longer have to worry about becoming personally engaged for a good decision. We can expect a pattern of automatic response to creep in: if there is a will, then there are no questions; if not, then we will have to clarify everything in discussions with the family members. Although the law provides for giving the family members an opportunity to voice their concerns, such a standardized approach threatens to become widespread because the modern market-oriented hospitals are ruled by economics and increasingly geared to acceleration. This means that fewer resources are kept available for the quiet discussion with the patients and their family members.

Lack of Confidence in the Humaneness of Modern Medicine?

Human beings are afraid of dying. And they are really afraid of dying in a hospital because they have found that many physicians are not easy to talk to when it comes to allowing death to come; rather, they are good technicians when it comes to preventing it. People try to overcome this fear with forms. In this setting, living wills can be seen as a shield that patients procure early to avoid the quagmire of the hospital "repair shop" that will otherwise seize control of them. In such a deficient health care system, the living will can indeed be necessary because whoever does not have one risks falling victim to the hospital machinery. And yet the question arises here of whether the living will is actually the right solution for the underlying problem.

Obviously such widespread use of living wills is due in no small measure to a lack of confidence in the humaneness of modern medicine. This lack of confidence cannot be addressed with a flood of forms.

146

The opposite is true: the more forms are filled out, the more preference will be given to a formalistic approach. And limiting everything to formal considerations strengthens the very reason why living wills became established in the first place, namely modern medicine's impersonal speechlessness and helplessness in dealing with these critical life issues. If the lack of confidence in medicine is indeed the reason behind many living wills, then the proper response on the part of modern medicine will be to invest in winning back this confidence.

The fundamental problem lies not in the lack of forms but in the lack of relationships, discussions, and time for the sick person, yet also in the lack of a certain fundamental attitude of being able to let go that future physicians hardly learn at all in medical school. If we look at this broader framework which has given rise to the debate about living wills, then it becomes clear that in places the living will is only a superficial cure that not only fails to solve but also actually exacerbates the underlying problem. This certainly does not apply to every living will. Yet if a large share of these wills are drafted because people are afraid, they will otherwise be robbed of their dignity in the hospital; then, the living will is nothing more than a suitable means of defending oneself within a bad system. A health care system that communicates awkwardly and is geared to mere expediency needs living wills to make the patient visible again. Yet is not such a situation more resigned than forward looking? The only thing that can be forward looking is to eliminate this deficient situation so that people no longer believe that as human beings they can only cope well with the hospital situation when they are armed with a living will. The more we emphasize living wills and ignore their larger context, the more we will witness an arms race with living wills within a health care system that inspires little confidence.

For a Culture of Dependence and Communicative Coexistence

In the discussions about living wills, mention is repeatedly made of situations in which following a living will should be understood as a demand to terminate all treatment.[63] However, such situations include more than just the "terminal" conditions in which technological means prevent an inevitable death. Often enough, it seems that merely the situation of being in need of help, of being dependent on others (see Chapter 6), of no longer being able to sufficiently provide for oneself is sufficient to request termination of treatment. My intention here is not to render a moral judgment on such expressions of will, nor is it to say that such expressions of will should not be followed. In a free society, one is obligated to respect every sort of refusal to undergo therapy.

> I feel it is important to reflect on why it is that people increasingly tend to see the mere condition of being dependent on other people as a sufficient reason to reject this life in every respect.

As long as living wills are recommended which express a rejection of any life that can only be lived with the aid of others, then this will entrench a tendency to fully depreciate life with sacrifices, to belittle life with disabilities, and to eliminate infirm life. If such wills become normality, then life in sickness will not be seen as life that requires particular care, rather increasingly as something that really does not have to be if one would only give freer rein to the patient's "autonomy." This is an expression of nothing less than an ideology of independence: life is only valued as long as the individual can subsist without dependence on the help of others. The moment he becomes infirm and dependent on others, his life automatically becomes something less than life. Veiled in a discussion of autonomy, a view is increasingly gaining ground in which only the independent self-sufficient person can lead a meaningful life. For all other life, the public generally finds it plausible to prefer death to life in infirmity.

People speak of autonomy, whereas they are essentially confusing autonomy with independence. They fail to recognize that one can retain one's autonomy even in the hours of greatest dependence by behaving toward this illness in one way or another. Humane medicine should ultimately advocate the understanding that dependence is not a defect but can be experienced as the starting point and an integral part of a humane health care system and world. Equating dependence on others to the "justified" termination of medical treatment as it is expressed in many living wills is sufficient cause for the health care system—as a social achievement—to become more involved with the patients in the future, to speak with the patients, and to demonstrate to them as experts for these disease conditions just how much potential lies dormant in people when they are in need of help.

Modern medicine's answer to many people's insidious fear of being at the mercy of others while dying must consist in offering trust and confidence—virtues that go well beyond what is discussed in the debate about living wills. Confidence can also come from knowing that modern medicine will have to honor the formal documents, and that is unquestionably a gain that the law has made possible. Yet it is necessary to treat living wills not as a checklist but to see in them a task of engaging more intensively with the patient and his environment. Merely following the living will in itself offers no guarantee of humane medicine. This will require promoting a new culture of dying, a culture that is realized every day and in every encounter with the patient, a new medicine that involves relationships and that sees the living will as part of a relationship and as a chance to enter a discussion about dying at a sufficiently early stage.

Chapter 8
Being Able to Let Go.
For a New Culture of Dying

Having to die is a basic existential experience for man. The prospect of death and the fear of suffering and transience shape our entire life. The advent of the dictate of feasibility has made us tend to comprehend even dying and death as something we can plan, as something whose time, nature, and conditions we would prefer to determine in advance. Active euthanasia—intentionally causing death—seems to be the appropriate answer here. But in rationalizing death are we not also losing the mystery of meaning? Can we live "well" when we suppress the finiteness of human existence? Can we die "well" when we do not succeed in becoming receptive for the greater context of life? This chapter will examine letting go and the mutual service that the living and the dying can perform for each other.

"Man is just a reed, nature's weakest, but he is a thinking reed. The entire universe need not arm itself to crush him; a vapor, a drop of water is enough to kill him. Yet if the universe crushed him then man would only be far nobler than that which kills him because he knows that he will die and what superiority the universe has over him. The universe knows nothing of this." (Blaise Pascal)

The thinking reed—that is man. From the outset he is vulnerable, from the outset liable to die at any time, but the fact that he knows that makes him something very special. Human life is a life of parting, it is a life in which departure is always present and which is permeated by departure. And yet today we do not really want to confront this. I recently came across an interview with an actress in the newspaper *Badische Zeitung* in which she admitted, "My bathroom is like a workshop. Every jar has 'repair' on it. I'm not afraid of getting old. Only death. I find it so superfluous, I could just explode. Yes, I would like to live forever."

It is entirely natural to fear death. It would be unfair to belittle the fear of death. It is also undoubtedly unacceptable to glorify the suffering connected with dying. Yet it is also wrong to leave it at this perspective of suffering. We must attempt to think further. My intuition tells me that suffering alone does not fully describe dying. The Austrian author Marie von Ebner-Eschenbach (1830–1916) put it in a nutshell: "The thought of the transience of all earthly things is a source of infinite suffering—and a source of infinite comfort." What is meant by this? How can this help us?

"Self-Determined Death"—Active Euthanasia Is Ethical Resignation

It is understandable that people wish to live with the greatest possible autonomy until the end of their life. Yet when this wish leads to an attitude of automatically regarding life as "deficient" or even "inhumane," once this autonomous control is no longer possible, then the legitimate wish becomes an ideological obsession. It is often suggested that dignity in death can only be preserved when control over the event is maintained. This fundamentally fails to acknowledge that dying is a phase of life that is characterized precisely by the fact that it escapes absolute controllability. Only if one frees oneself of the desire to have everything under control even when dying will one become capable of accepting death as a part of life.

The way in which the media reported how Gunter Sachs ended his life after diagnosing himself with Alzheimer's disease has given me pause. A person kills himself and the media report almost euphorically about a struggle for his own death, even a death with dignity—and hardly anyone appears shocked. And I asked myself how can it be that we have apparently forgotten how to react appropriately to a suicide? How can it be that we are no longer shaken when we hear that a person who actually could have lived longer came to the conclusion that nonexistence is preferable to existence in our society? A society that does not react to a suicide with shock but declares it to be an understandable death runs the risk of sending others to their death because this indicates that our society can find suicide plausible and reasonable. A society that finds it reasonable when one takes one's own life in the face of a disease is dangerous. Because more than ever it will drive many struggling people to despair who doubt that their life still has value and wonder whether they have only become a burden.

Books advocating active euthanasia and propagating assisted suicide have become bestsellers because they appear to give an answer to the fear and suffering from the transience of life. They have also become bestsellers because they confirm and strengthen a dominant mindset of our age, namely the thinking that a life that can no longer be lived "autonomously" is a worthless life. That's the reason for the call for assisted suicide, for active euthanasia, and also for termination of therapy even in the absence of a terminal condition (the last hours or days of life).

> We differentiate four types of euthanasia:
> * Passive euthanasia: refusal, reduction, or termination of medical therapy in a severely ill patient.

- *Indirect euthanasia: medical treatment of a condition of suffering that accepts the risk of shortening the patient's life.*
- *Active euthanasia: consciously and intentionally causing death at the express wish of the patient.*
- *Assisted suicide: aiding the patient in killing himself.*

In a 2006 position paper on end-of-life care, the German Ethics Council recommended a departure from the distinction between passive and active euthanasia and instead advocated differentiation in (1) end-of-life care, (2) hospice care, (3) allowing to die, (4) assisted suicide, and (5) killing on request.

"My Death Is My Own"

Today, autonomy is commonly understood as individual self-determination in the sense that the will of an individual becomes binding once someone decides something for himself without harming others. This emancipated self-determination should apply in every phase of life, including the phase of sickness and dying. Yet I ask myself: Must not the situation in which the wish to die arises be considered an exceptional situation? In other words, can such a demand for autonomy be at all appropriate for the situation of dying as a situation of extreme weakness and occasionally even of despair and resignation? Might not the demand for autonomous determination be too abstract for the situation of extreme distress in which people who prefer not to live any longer find themselves?

These questions are significant insofar as many people regard it as a "compulsion to live" when they are refused the right to determine the time of their death as autonomously as possible. This is apparently the reason for the broad support that active euthanasia enjoys. Many people regard it as unacceptable paternalism when their demand to have themselves killed is not followed. But let us look at this more closely: Can we really speak of a "compulsion to live" here? Is it not true that one can only be forced into something when there is something to choose but one is not allowed to choose? As I see it, this brings us to the key question underlying the discussion about active euthanasia. It pertains only superficially to individual self-determination. In fact, what is being debated here is whether life is given and therefore immutable or whether it is made and as such is at our free disposal.

> Whoever speaks about the compulsion to live in connection with the prohibition of active euthanasia implicitly assumes that life is not something given but an option, indeed the result of a personal decision.

Why is this veiled connection between the assertion of a right to autonomous self-determination and the view that our life is something that we, with legal authorization, can end or have ended when we so desire so crucial? It is crucial because in a certain way it runs counter to the question posed at the beginning as to whether the situation in which the wish to die arises must be considered an exceptional situation. If a person's autonomy is defined so broadly that even the person's own life is at his disposal, then we really do not have to worry any more about whether there are other ways to deal with this exceptional situation, to accompany the person through this situation, and thus mitigate it. If the dying person's "autonomy" is of penultimate importance at every minute of his living and dying, then the thought of care is secondary. The danger that the decision of the person wanting to die arises from his situation of extreme desperation then becomes, as Udo Reiter expressed in his plea "My Death Is My Own" in the *Süddeutsche Zeitung*, a "risk" that is "inextricably bound to a free society" and the possible "wrong decision" that we extinguish the life of an individual in despair of his life instead of helping him becomes a "consequence of freedom."[64]

"Preventing Unnecessary Suffering"

In addition to autonomy, a second argument is commonly used to support active euthanasia, and that is that unnecessary suffering can be prevented with active euthanasia. However, this argumentation requires us to think carefully about how we can define suffering. Suffering is ultimately defined by the human experience of loss; a person suffers from an experience that conflicts with his own view of a good life. What is seen as a loss and what is seen as intolerable suffering depends decisively on each individual person's attitude to life. Thus, suffering is only intolerable when the individual defines it as intolerable with respect to his or her personal life goals. With the exception of extreme physical pain, there is no generally acceptable definition of "intolerable suffering."

As "intolerable suffering" ultimately depends on the attitude and not on the situation as such, an appropriate response on the part of the physician would appear to me to consist in helping the patient not to see life as futile despite the most severe limitation. In the face of all difficulties, the task of the healing professions in particular in these difficult situations must be to point out prospects, however slight they may be. If one assumes that "suffering" is defined in the context of a certain understanding of a "good life," then an appropriate treatment of suffering in the setting of an incurable disease should be sought in offering the patient help in integrating the disease into his view of a good life instead of extinguishing the patient himself. Or, in other words, if one proceeds with the assumption that the extent of suffering depends on the image of a life without suffering, then does it not seem plausible to work on this image instead of destroying the life?

Dying Means Being Able to Let Go

The fiction of being able to maintain life in total independence until the end seems to me to be more of a risk to the good life. For it ignores the simple fact that a human being is a dependent entity from the outset and throughout his entire existence. The modern tendency to interpret being dependent on other people as the end of autonomy can only be regarded as an expression of suppression of the human condition that implies nothing other than the fear of being rendered powerless, losing control, and having to let go. Our society would not like to admit this fear and reinterprets it as the pathos of freedom. Yet it overlooks the fact that genuine freedom really consists in first accepting the essential characteristics of being human and then realizing that in light of one's own frailty one can only remain oneself by learning to let go, to let go of the fiction that one should never be dependent on other people throughout one's entire life.

> Sooner or later every one of us will have to let go and put ourselves in other people's hands because there is no dying without letting go.

Whoever categorically refuses these hands and prefers to end life sooner sacrifices himself to a life-denying control imperative.

The experience of hospice caregivers and palliative medicine in particular has repeatedly shown that the wish to die in the setting of a severe illness should usually be seen as a transitory phase, an initial resignation, a shock in the face of lost prospects. If we only show this person the way to assisted suicide, we overlook the fact that this

157

transitory phase can also be overcome with a culture of consolation and care. The key task of society should accordingly be to give something back to people who initially despair in the face of their illness, something which has been completely neglected in the current discussion about euthanasia: confidence, comfort, and showing how one can tap one's own existing resources. As long as a life exists, it is like a light. One needs to only open one's eyes for this light that is still shining.

Today, we tend to and want to have everything under control, yet we fail to see that an appropriate way of dealing with death can include seeing it as fate, as an experience that begins to make sense for the very reason that it is—luckily—beyond the absolute control of human beings. In many other eras, the manner and time of death were seen as something that man has no right to influence. Yet today not only life but also dying is commonly seen as something that man no longer need anticipate but must bring about himself. This is often seen as increased freedom. What is ignored is that this wish to exercise influence can also mean an enormous loss and an enormous burden.

The Rationalization of Death and the Question of "Meaning"

My main criticism of the current debates about euthanasia thus pertains to the fundamental attitudes underlying the pleas for "self-determined" death. In all of these debates, dying and death are no longer understood as modalities of human existence. On the contrary, we only seem to see deficient aspect of them, which then should no longer be at all. Dying is not seen as the consummation of life but only as the zero state of being human. And because it is seen in this way, people wish death to be gone, and with it dying. Accordingly, many debates are not about good dying, but about banishing it completely. Because dying does not seem to fit in with life, people do not see why they should have to wait for death either. It would be better to bring about death oneself according to one's own criteria than to wait for it, so the credo goes. I feel that the attitude of anticipating, waiting, and accepting can be an appropriate way of dealing with dying as a part of life, and not the attitude of doing.

Yet waiting for one's own death to mature within life seems to be irreconcilable with current tendencies to accelerate the pace of life. Hyperactivity, multitasking, and keeping multiple options open—none of this is really compatible with being able to wait patiently. The modern fundamental attitudes of rationalism and activism cause us to want to determine and plan in advance the type of our death, its circumstances, and its time. The effect of this is nothing else than distancing ourselves from the incomprehensibility of death. The intent is to remove the mysterious and hidden aspect from death—the intangible—by placing it under the control of planning. And does this not also indicate a tendency to secularize and trivialize it? In any case, modern man cannot simply let death approach him; he wants to take control of it. As important as it undoubtedly is not to face death entirely unprepared and as essential as it is to support the dying person in doing so, death cannot simply be planned like a project. The more we attempt to take control of it, the more we blind ourselves to the insight that death will always have something mysterious about it.

The end of life eludes our control just as much as its beginning for the very reason that we cannot objectify death but ultimately can "only" suffer it.

We have to allow the impossibility of complete objectification of death to sink in, and we must admit to ourselves that death, like life, remains an indeterminable mystery. Only then will we be in a position to deal with death prudently. This also has something to do with "meaning" because meaning always has something indeterminate about it. Meaning can and may remain indeterminate, even vague. It allows room for what is intangible, for what is indeterminable, for mystery— mystery not in the sense of not yet knowing, but in the sense of fundamentally never being able to know. For the mystery has nothing to do with magic, but has to do with spirituality.

Spirituality Is an Orientation toward the Question of Meaning

With this reference to spirituality, we touch upon a level of the human being that is incontestably integral to coming to terms with the crisis situation brought on by dying. To this extent, spirituality is a very important aspect of the dying person's being a person, and anyone who ignores this key aspect does not entirely do justice to the human being as such. We can only maintain this as long as we understand spirituality to be something very general, namely an indelible aspect of the human being. I do not mean solely the specific experience of faith, the religious conviction. I would understand "spirituality" far more generally and fundamentally as an orientation toward the question of meaning, occasionally also in the form of experiencing meaning. In any case, I would understand it as a relationship to the world that transcends what is merely purposeful because the orientation toward purposes alone would mean that one would jump from one purpose to the next and would inevitably become caught in a thicket of purposes without being able to say exactly to what end all of them are ultimately good. Spirituality understood in this sense would thus be a desire to go beyond oneself, a "transcending of the limits of one's own givenness as self and opening to a larger and more powerful reality which is different from the materiality and contingency of what is merely present."[65] This element of transcending what is merely materially present into a sphere of the spirit places one's own self in a larger context. For this reason, spirituality is often, although not necessarily, associated with a longing for unity. The modern tendency to rationalize dying ignores man's spiritual endowment by attempting to make this mysterious larger context accessible to technology and programmable. In so doing, it does justice neither to the dying person nor to dying in principle.

Spirituality not only fulfills a fundamental need on the part of human beings to follow goals, but also can endow meaning in and of itself by freeing man from self-centeredness. This liberation is all the more beneficial given that one must recognize that ultimately "the human being completely on his own who seeks the meaning of his life exclusively within himself is condemned to fail in his effort to find fulfillment in his existence."[66] According to the psychotherapist Robert F. Antoch, one way of endowing with meaning by overcoming self-centeredness arises from the recognition of selfhood in relatedness. With this notion, Antoch harkens back to the founder of individual psychology Alfred Adler (1870–1937) who indicated how much man is capable of a "sense of community" with the world, from which the mutual conditionality of individual and community clearly follows. Spirituality in the sense outlined earlier, namely, as an orientation toward the question of meaning, could, accordingly, be understood as a step toward a capacity for relationship, as a spiritual way of establishing a relationship to the community and to the world. In line with Adler, it could be said that spirituality can lead to the conviction that every human being has ultimately received everything that he is from the community and that he as a human being continues to draw on what is communal and can draw on it in shaping his life and his dying. From this sense of community flows the feeling of gratitude that should be regarded as a power in itself. Gratitude for what is given, for what was already there without one's own effort, for what one is: a given being to whose givenness one has contributed nothing oneself. Thus, it is gratitude in the sense of perceiving this fundamental condition of "owing."

The "Private" Death and the Community

In addition to the modern tendency to rationalize dying, there is increasingly a tendency to privatize it. Death has thus largely mutated into what is now only an individualized event. If we can no longer regard death as a part of something communal but only as "one's own" death (and thus also the death of what is one's own), then we have removed death from its social bonds, removed it from the world of the community. It has been released into the private realm precisely because it is no longer regarded as part of a culture but as a product of what is mine.

Naturally, it is a key point that each person dies in his own way. Martin Heidegger introduced the concept of the "discrete mineness" (Jemeinigkeit) of death, and in the writings of Rainer Maria Rilke, we also find the notion that everyone should "be able to die his own death" vividly presented. Nonetheless, we must not fail to recognize that even and especially one's own individual death requires a community that provides stability, a community that represents what we may call the enabling condition for one's own death. In the past, it was the social and religious norms that provided support through the self-evident presence of a social community, and despite all the attendant pressure to conform never released the person into isolation. Death was also a social event.[67] Today death is supposed to be a completely private individual event, and yet we sense that without a community, without a person opposite us, we cannot die well.

The French philosopher Paul Ricoeur (1913–2005), in his notes published posthumously under the title *Living Up To Death*, expressly addressed "having to die that is common to all." He sees having to die as something that we not only all share but in which we can gain a fundamental meaning for each other, by accompanying each other through it. To succor the dying person instead of merely "surviving" him, to participate in his dying as he precedes us instead of merely seeing him from the outside as a disappearing life—according to Ricoeur it is only in this manner that we do justice to the dying person in his dying as a consummation of life. Thus, the experience of death, when we confront it, necessarily runs through the community, through the person opposite, the other, and because of this it also acquires a consoling dimension. It is true that at the moment of death each must die "his own" separate death. *Yet he does not die it alone.* In other words, his dying is not characterized solely by "isolation," but by a community of fellow human beings that stands in solidarity and thus by a sort of "resurrection," as Ricoeur says, in the community of the living.

I regard palliative medicine and hospice work as a necessary and beneficial counterpoint to the individualizing tendencies of the modern age because hospice work can create a new social community. A community with the hospice workers but also with the family members, the neighbors, and the various professional groups who themselves form a community. An important purpose of paid and voluntary hospice work thus consists in creating a community with the dying, because it is only through such a community that dying is not merely accepted but is turned back to life and the living. Turned back not in the sense of a prolongation of life but in the sense of an intensification of life, of allowing "experiencing life" in dying. Must not, as Ricoeur also asks, life in the face of dying be written in capital letters, because here it is present in its greatest density, in its fundamental mystery?[68]

Being Able to Accept One's Life

What is important in dealing with and accompanying dying people? A helper's answer to this "exceptional situation," as the German psychiatrist and philosopher Karl Jaspers (1883–1969) called it, can only be a "comprehensive" one, namely the answer of a person, an entire human being, and not the answer of a proficient service provider. Even today we should understand medicine as caritas, which as the original Latin word suggests, is a love of one's neighbor arising from appreciation, as care in the service of the other. This care for the sick person can become a help for the other person if it becomes help in overcoming something. Help in overcoming a life crisis, which dying can but need not necessarily represent.

The dying person may go through a crisis because his view of his life has become so painfully clear and the recognition of what is irretrievable, of a life that has happened once and for all, can be very painful. Such a dying person needs someone at his side who might again move him to become receptive for the value of what is past and for the value of a life waning yet still existing, for the flame of life that is becoming smaller and casting longer shadows yet still burns and gives light. Dying is often associated with suffering. But it is not suffering from pain alone, which can usually be treated, but primarily from that which is past and irretrievably gone, from a life whose past is immutable and whose future is becoming ever shorter. The dying that is approaching means having to accept that to an ever-increasing degree one has already lived and nearly all the cards have been played.

Dying is ultimately a sort of test of whether one succeeds in accepting the life one has lived oneself as such.

Dying is a test of whether or not one can accept one's own life story. The more genuine and fulfilled the life was, the easier it will be to die because it is easier to accept what is irretrievably gone. Yet a life that was lived missing the point of life is particularly painful in the face of having to die because one only has a very limited second chance. And this is precisely where care for the dying person acquires a special meaning. Care that might possibly be able to make it clear that every life necessarily remains fragmented and that one's own life, despite being fragmented and imperfect, might have a deeper meaning. Care that can consist in helping the suffering person to find peace—with himself and with the life he has lived.

In this setting, we must remind ourselves that the benefit of end-of-life care can consist precisely in the fact that the encounter with a helper gives rise to a new strength for the dying person, the strength to see the things of the world and his own life differently than before. This new strength of seeing the world differently would be something like a deeper "therapy" that ultimately becomes for that very reason a genuine support in life and makes possible an attitude of acceptance with respect to oneself and the world. One could see such a "therapy" as an aid to accepting one's own limitation and to accepting the world as it is and oneself. Caring for dying people in a deeper sense could mean helping put the patient in a good relationship to his own life, his sickness, and his dying. That would also mean helping the dying person not to simply exclude the process of dying by means of assisted suicide, active euthanasia, or appropriate living wills but to overcome it himself.

What Could Good Dying Look Like?

Having to die is not merely a form of death crisis; it is a form of life crisis. Dying recalls the life that one has lived and that cannot be lived again. In this crisis, one must give the patient hope and confidence. Having hope means being rendered able to make peace with this past life in order to achieve the confidence that everything will be fine. Accepting the past life that cannot be relived would be the way to overcome the suffering from having to die. The dying person needs a person opposite him who makes him receptive for this dimension. Even in the face of having to die, there is still a chance, there is still a good way there, there is still a good that can accompany this dying. This is the fundamental hope directed toward a saving word. This is a word that helps the person know he is still supported, the word that is still able to carry the person even in the face of a narrowed horizon, that continues to bring him further along in his life. It is ultimately about a word that the person can rely on, that exudes trust, that speaks trust. Therefore, we can say that a decisive characteristic of hope for the human being is this hoping for a word.

A key task of end-of-life care, as I see it, would have to lie in making the dying person receptive for what may be a long buried feeling of gratitude for life itself. Were one to succeed in making room for this fundamental feeling, one would have achieved everything it is possible to achieve in caring for the other because this feeling of gratitude changes everything else. The dying person then experiences a tranquility that is more inward than outward, a satisfaction with the world, and an acceptance of what has past. One cannot prescribe this acceptance, but one can help the dying person again become receptive for it.

Overcoming Self-Centeredness

Dying can only be overcome when the person succeeds in largely freeing himself from control and from the dictate of wanting to do and dispose and becomes receptive to the insight that dying cannot be adequately encountered in the attitude of doing. Precisely at the end of life it becomes clear as never before that each of us comes to life only by way of many determinants and that we return again by way of just such determinants. Neither we can say that we have made the world into which we were born, nor can we say that we "make" our end.

> Dying illustrates man's connection with a greater framework from which he comes and into which he is again released in some form. Recognizing and accepting this framework seems to me to be very important for dying well.

Yet precisely in dying something else becomes clearer than ever before: that the life that is reaching its end is something every human being has simply received. He simply received life as a gift. He did not choose it and did not make it. He did nothing for the fact that he exists. He is a human being who fundamentally owes his life. And when one realizes this, then it will become clear that life is nothing less than a gift. This thought can be very consoling because it can free one from claims to this life, even if it is the claim to wanting to live longer or to determine the end oneself. If life has been given as a gift, then the appropriate way to deal with it and the reaction to this life is not the attitude of entitlement but that of gratitude that it exists at all.

Proceeding from this "brightening gratitude," Paul Ricoeur goes a step further in his thinking. He turns the service performed by the person accompanying the dying person performed into a service that now proceeds from the dying person and that has something to do with this gratitude received "in the face of what is essential." The receptiveness for what is essential that bursts open in the threshold experience of dying allows the life that has become concentrated in the dying person to flow back into the other in a certain sense; it itself becomes a gift that the dying person gives to the person at his side and in whose company he may die his death. In this way, as Ricoeur writes, one could understand the act of dying in a deeper sense as an act of life, as a mutual "service to the other."[69]

On the Significance of Serenity at the End of Life

In light of these considerations, I advocate a new respect for serenity, especially in dealing with dying. I do not mean serenity in the sense of passivity, but in the sense of grateful acceptance of what is given, of the gift. The limitation of life is something given and in it lies a great opportunity to experience meaning or the "essential," as Ricoeur calls it. Without the limitation of life, one could not give any meaning to life because the possible infiniteness of life would render it impossible for man to shape his life meaningfully. If we lived forever, we could just as easily do what we wanted to do today a hundred years from now. Why today? Why now?

To this extent, the fact that we have to die is not a tragedy but our salvation. The philosopher Martin Heidegger put it in a nutshell: death is the before-state of life. It is always present and only in the awareness of death are we required to shape our life and take care of it. Having to die is thus not a realm of our later years but a basic hallmark of our entire life. And the more we bear in mind that we have to die, the more consciously we will be able to live.

Not only the finiteness of life but also the uncertainty of the time of our death is given. *Mors certa, hora incerta* is the saying: every person's death is as certain as its hour is uncertain. What a blessing this uncertainty is! Precisely because we know that we will die but do not know exactly when; we can use this uncertainty as the basis for both hoping and waiting. What we fail to see in this age of management is that it is the openness of life, the uncertainty about the future that can give our lives meaning. If we knew exactly what would happen tomorrow, if everything went according to our plan, then this life would lose its meaning. We would only have the feeling of being the executor of a plan but not the feeling of genuinely shaping our life. For we only feel ourselves as its shaper when life produces something unexpected, when it is strewn with what is unpredictable and imponderable, when it is full of events that surprise us. Even what is unsolicited belongs to those things in life that give it depth and give us the chance to reveal ourselves as the shapers of our life. Faced with what we can neither avert nor alter, we can still remain ourselves: we ourselves who find our own way to deal with what is unsolicited and to grasp it in a way that only we can, and in so doing realize ourselves.

The freedom that we as human beings have is not realized in executing a preordained plan but precisely in confronting what we have not chosen for ourselves.

> We regard ourselves as free human beings precisely when we have the feeling that we have proven ourselves in an encounter we never would have chosen.

Certainly, the point is not to glorify what is unsolicited. What is unsolicited is unsolicited and as such it would be better if we did not have it. Yet a life in which we did not have anything unsolicited, in which we were neither challenged nor surprised nor faced with a task to solve, would probably be an entirely meaningless life. For what should we do with it? I am fully aware that this a very thin line: When is the unsolicited a threat and when is it an opportunity? And yet we often overlook our resources, we overlook how much we have received in the way of deep inner reserves which we need only mobilize and have the courage to use. Viktor Frankl (1905–1997), the Austrian psychiatrist and concentration camp survivor, made it abundantly clear to us that suffering in itself will not crush a human being, but only meaningless suffering.

Yet precisely in dealing with dying it is not what is unsolicited that saves us, but the uncertainty. Not knowing when. Many people today no longer want to wait for an uncertain hour but want to determine when and how they will die. They do not want to resign themselves to what is given but want to take their time of death into their own hands and shape it. I have experienced many patients with amyotrophic lateral sclerosis (ALS), a degenerative disease of the motor nervous system, who decided that they would rather die than have to be put on a respirator. They could have determined the time of their death themselves yet many of them ultimately shied away from doing so because they had doubts about whether it was really the right time, whether it might be too early. Many kept postponing the planned time of death until death finally came of its own accord. What I am trying to say is this: today we may not want to accept what is given, we want to shape things, but this shaping and determining oneself can also be a great burden. Therefore, it seems to me that the fundamental attitude of serenity, of expectation, is appropriate for dying, especially since only this attitude can offer the opportunity of maturing to the process of dying so to speak, and of not squaring up with this life but rounding it off.

Of course, every person is unique and has his very own goals. Therefore, it is important even in the final phase of life to create spaces to allow every person to die in his own way: spaces for a person's own death, which does not necessarily mean a death alone. Help for dying people can only be realized if we regard them as unique people who have great potential even in the final phase of their life. The task should be in every discussion to find this specific potential and make the infirm person receptive for the insight that there can never be a state in which it is completely absent. Help for people at the end of life therefore means above all ensuring that a culture of dying arises that is replete with fellow human beings giving comfort and confidence who have a good relationship with the dying person. Ultimately, it is not being able to do something, but a person's confidence in a community of fellow human beings that is the greatest comfort and thus the best basis for dying in dignity.

For the final task of medicine, like all social professions, is not making and producing health, not the manufacture of a life without suffering, but the promise of being there when "there is nothing more to be done," because it is precisely then that what is truly essential can be "done": filling the remaining lifespan with a life-affirming fundamental attitude. Precisely that is what I see as the core virtue of the physician, which can be nothing else than one of love for the patient that gives of oneself. Therein lies the greatest gift that one can give a dying person: helping the patient by means of appreciative attention to say yes to his own life and to do this even in his weakest and final hour.

Epilogue: Happiness Lies in Our Attitude toward the World

Now, we have spanned a broad range of topics and touched upon man's core existential questions, and we have kept encountering the basic question: Do we really want what we are able to do? We have repeatedly come to the point where it has become clear to us that what initially looked like a beneficial case of overcoming a limitation, upon closer inspection, revealed the danger of us becoming prisoners of what is feasible. What at first seemed to be liberation from the shackles of nature often revealed itself to be compulsion to follow a new dictate, namely the dictate of social expectation—in no small measure the expectation that what is possible will also be realized. And yet to simply issue a blanket condemnation of these expansions of our frontiers that technology and science has made possible would be a cheap criticism indeed. Most of us owe our health, often even our lives, to precisely this technology and to the scientific approach to man that medicine teaches. Thus, the solution to the problems cannot be a blanket criticism of feasibility. Rather, it is a matter of critically and discriminatingly learning to differentiate what liberates us from what enslaves us. Up to what point do these options help us to achieve a freer and more fulfilled life? At what point do they no longer do so, but begin to exert control over us? Therefore, this book will conclude not with destructive criticism but with constructive ethics, namely the ethics of prudence.

Medicine of Prudence

In answer to my criticism of a medicine without measure, which only knows doing, does not pause, and has no understanding for the sense of a limit, I have proposed prudence as a solution and as a guideline for the problems I have outlined. When we hear prudence, we may think of contemplation, of doing nothing, of hesitating. The opposite is true. The concept of prudence was used by Homer as the opposite of hubris ("excessive self-confidence"); the original Greek sophrosyne meant nothing other than "healthy sense." Plato described prudence as "harmony of the whole" and as "health of the soul." Arthur Schopenhauer (1788–1860) provided the most accurate description when he emphasizes that prudence consists in the ability to step back from the moment and "to survey the entirety of life."

Above all, three aspects of prudence are important for the topics in this book:
1. Prudence requires intelligence and realism. That means one must recognize the realities as they are. A prudent person is not a dreamer. He does not imagine the world as it should be without simultaneously relating to the world of which he is a part. That means that realism is an essential condition for prudent decisions. However, realism does not mean that one quickly puts up with what is. I think a prudent person acknowledges reality without accepting it as inalterable. That is the crux of the matter. The prudent person is a person with confidence, namely the confidence that it is worthwhile to advocate changing reality and to believe that what exists today must not remain so forever. It is a confidence such that he does not struggle with what exists and succumb to the feeling of his own powerlessness, but in his sharp view of reality perceives the opportunity of using its current state

as the point of departure for a change—even if this change is only in his own attitude to this reality. It is up to us whether we accept reality resignedly and in so doing further cement it or whether we grasp it as a point of departure and an opportunity to realize ourselves in the face of this reality by shaping it and thus gradually changing it.

> A key characteristic of prudence is that it can produce a harmony between what is and what ideally could be.

2. In addition to realism, an inner calm is another essential condition for prudence. It is important that a person not let himself be carried away by the offers and promises without assuming a contemplative attitude toward them. Prudence means that one does not allow oneself to be steamrollered by developments; rather, it means that one counters their apparent intrinsic logic with the power of reflection to keep them under control. Whoever reflects is not simply opposed to a development but ponders it calmly. He does not merely weigh benefits and risks but also the question of what the new entity means for his own self-image. It is not a matter of doing a calculation. On the contrary, a prudent person is one who understands how to question the goals himself, that is, someone who focuses his reflection precisely on the fundamental and nonquantitative aspects of the question. Applied to us, we can ultimately understand prudence as a prerequisite for selfhood, for a reflective selfhood insofar as it keeps us from thoughtlessly relinquishing our own authenticity. Yet it is not merely calmness in thinking, that is to say not merely an intellectual virtue; rather, prudence invariably means a virtue of character as well: the virtue of steadfastness and of "inner

superiority." This means it is necessary that one develop an understanding of oneself that prevents one from being immoderate in one's own demands on life and that prevents one from being immoderate in one's own emotions. A prudent person has learned to avoid being overcome by these emotions because he knows that can cause him to see the world one-sidedly and possibly make decisions that could prove to be too shortsighted.

Prudence implies moderation with emotions; it implies finding proportion in the emotions of fear but also hope, finding proportion in the emotions of longing but also worry.

3. Prudence requires a desire to act. That is crucial. Precisely the semantic proximity of prudence to the concept of contemplation could tempt us to misunderstand the ethics of prudence as a matter of accepting everything as it is and simply suppressing the inner drive to change something. That would be a totally incorrect understanding of prudence. On the contrary, a prudent person is one who is determined to take action—not upon his first impulse, but after an adequate period of reflection. He is a person who decides for himself, who can decide to take this or that action. Someone who simply exercises forbearance may be serene (and that is very valuable) but he is not automatically prudent. Prudence recognizes the goals that are worthy of taking action to pursue, and it realizes itself when this differentiation is followed by a decision and with that decision the steadfast will to put into practice what has been decided. Thus, an ethics of prudence always attempts to see the whole and demands that one strive with respect to the whole for the realization of the recognizable good in the sense of the good life.

Maybe one could illustrate the ethics of prudence by using an analogy to a bird that has always been regarded as the very symbol of prudence: the owl. The owl has such large and highly developed eyes that it can see things that remain hidden to other animals. As it has a field of binocular vision of 70 degrees, it can see nearly everywhere. The owl can turn its head up to 270 degrees, giving it astounding flexibility and adaptability. The owl's eyes are everywhere; they see the whole world. And they see the whole world at night because their giant cornea gives them this ability. They also have exceptional hearing and can immediately pinpoint the source of any sound however fast it may be moving. When one observes owls, one is impressed by the great calm and patience that they exhibit even when hunting. If we now consider this capacity in a symbolic sense, we could say that the owl symbolizes sharp-sightedness and foresight, even when it has become dark all around. That means when everyone else has lost their way or when everyone in this intellectual darkness follows what everyone else follows or follows what is most comfortable or closest, whether it be habit or the ideology of one's own age, the way of thinking that one is used to.

With respect to the existential questions we have examined in this book, we can ultimately say that a person can only become happy if he succeeds in developing an inner superiority with respect to all the options of modern medicine that prevents him from being drawn into the feasibility quagmire. The quagmire created by the technological options nullifies prudence, for, once one is caught in the quagmire, one usually no longer notices how one step leads to the next. Everything appears so natural that we fall into patterns of automatic response that we no longer shape by reflection. Instead, we ourselves are shaped as if by an invisible law and are swept along in a direction that we never would have consciously chosen. Remaining prudent as a physician and as a patient means nothing other than being able to keep from being blinded by the arsenal of options and instead to see the enticements of an increasingly market-driven medical industry in proper perspective.

Where Is the Yardstick?

Medicine without a sense of proportion was the diagnosis I made. A medicine with a sense of proportion can only exist in a society that itself has lost its sense of proportion. What has to be done now? It is important to remember that man is the only animal that must find his sense of proportion himself. Animals do not know excess; they are guided only by their instincts. Man can be seduced and led astray, seduced by promises, seduced by the consumerist logic of constant increase. Unlike animals, man does not simply find his yardstick in nature because man's nature ultimately consists in being able to and having to transcend his own nature with reason. Therefore, the suggestion occasionally made in light of today's skewed developments that man should find his way back to his nature is not entirely logical. Man is a being that is called upon to use his reason. He is called upon to open up new horizons because that is an integral part of his nature. What would man be if he had not always refined the instruments of his reason, right down to the art of writing as one of his salient cultural achievements?

It is not the transcending nature that is the problem but identifying the limit beyond which further transcendence would cease to be in keeping with his nature as a human being. Finding this limit represents a new challenge for every epoch and every culture because it cannot be found in nature but only in the mind of man. Nor can this limit be pinned down once and for all; it must be created anew in every epoch, creatively developed anew, because every epoch has new

177

challenges to overcome and in every epoch man must gaze on new horizons. In this setting, the answer to our question cannot be back to nature, back to fatalism, or back to earlier times. We need solutions for the future that cannot simply be copied from the past. Yet, the past, the traditions which we have grown out of, can help us to better find our way. For the history of our thought is full of fascinating insights and guides to a good life. Many of them we have touched on in the past chapters and a few of them we have even examined in greater detail. Now let us apply the question of a good life to medicine and ask: What can an ethics of prudence mean for modern medicine, and how can modern medicine contribute to people being able to lead a good life?

Medicine and the Question of the Good Life

I feel one fundamental problem that runs through every chapter lies in the fact that modern medicine nearly invariably reacts with hyper-activity, with the promise of what is feasible, the vision of altering the body. It has always responded in a way that reduces the body to an object and "machines" it one way or another. A medicine fixated on feasibility invariably relies on tweaking the external circumstances of life; it relies on correcting the sick body. However, it ignores the fact that man's freedom extends beyond shaping the external manifestations. Man's greatest freedom consists in the choice of his inner attitude toward the given external circumstances. We live in an era characterized by the attitude that there is nothing we have to put up with, and thus the modern world designs entire arsenals for conquering the world.

The credo that the world should fundamentally be conquered and not accepted is one that paralyzes the great resources that man has when he works not only on the external world but also on his inner attitude to the world.

Here it can be beneficial to recall what is, in its simple givenness. In this way, every human being can be rendered capable of encountering what exists with a fundamental attitude of acceptance. Accepting what is—that is the key resource that every human being should learn to fall back on. For only in this attitude of acceptance will he be rendered able to deal constructively with his limits.

Let us use a severe illness as an example. Medicine has taught us to see the healthy, able-bodied person as the guiding principle and to emphasize the deficiencies in someone that does not live up to this guiding principle. Yes, medicine has taught us to see being ill as a malfunction that one should fear as a catastrophe. The guiding principle of the invariably able-bodied person is a problematic point of departure for a humane medicine because it cannot regard sick and dependent people as a malfunction. On the contrary, the physician will only be able to really help the sick person if becoming sick is seen as an intrinsic characteristic of human beings, indeed recognized as a form of human existence. Only when being able to become sick is accepted as an intrinsic characteristic of human beings is it possible to react to this form of existence with a fundamental attitude of understanding, with a fundamental attitude that can first accept this state of existence as it is. Only this attitude of being able to let something stand as it is and to avoid comparing it to a fictitious ideal makes it possible to find meaning in this state of existence. Namely, meaning that allows the person to integrate the new experience of being sick into his own life. This integrating of the physical change due to sickness into one's own life naturally includes appropriate medical treatment of the change. Yet it can help prevent treating and "fighting" the illness from becoming an obsession with the consequence that the person who has become sick overlooks the fact that he can lead a more fulfilled life even as a "weak" and dependent person. The possibility of leading a fulfilled life in sickness is one that modern man forbids himself. This is not because of the sickness itself but primarily because of a problematic self-interpretation that leads many people to experience their becoming sick only with an attitude of "fighting" it.

Let me illustrate this point with an example from ancient times: The Stoic school of philosophy used the image of the "leash of fate" for the fate of man. It is like a dog tied to a moving wagon. The leash allows the dog a lot of freedom of movement but not unlimited freedom. It is ultimately the leash of fate that leads him. This image may seem to us today to be too narrow, yet it also has a timeless message. The dog can move completely freely within its radius. If it does not accept the leash at all and wants to be completely free, that means if it constantly fights the leash, then it will ultimately lose even the freedom to move as it pleases within the space allotted to it. This is how Seneca should be understood when he emphasizes in his letter to Lucilius, "Fate leads the willing, and drags along the reluctant." Modern man and modern medicine react to fate as the reluctant one whom fate then drags along. Modern medicine occasionally leads people to believe they could be rid of the leash entirely and in many cases makes them less free than they were before because with its medical promise it robs them of the opportunity to move freely within their radius. Medicine wants to hear nothing of the value of accepting oneself because it itself has fallen victim to a delusion of feasibility and knows only change and no pause, only activism and no contemplation, because, in the words of the philosopher Hans Blumenberg, it has succumbed to the "sedative of dynamism." This is all the more tragic for medicine because it renders it unable to fulfill its task of helping people.

The Chance of Inner Healing Power

It is time for medicine to depart from its one-sided concentration on technological feasibility and turn to the sick person as a healing science that renders him receptive to his intrinsic capability to overcome what is unavoidable fate by accepting it as a part of his own life. Only then would it comprehensively do justice to the sick person because it is a fundamental human need to ask the question of meaning and to pursue goals. A person can do nothing other than ask the question of meaning, and this is all the more true in the face of suffering caused by illness. Therefore, it is a key task of medicine to help people find meaning from within themselves. Naturally it is not possible to see becoming sick simply as meaningful. Being sick is always something not desired, something obstructive that one would prefer not to have to suffer. Yet when it is present, immutably present, then every person has the opportunity to react to the sickness in such a manner that it does not remain completely meaningless. The sickness can be a vital indication of the vulnerable points of a person's life. Sickness brings a person into exceptional situations and it is often what shows him that ultimately every person has received everything that he is from some ultimate source. He did not make himself, he did not choose and want his life. It was simply given to him. All of life is simply a gift and only this givenness makes it possible for a human being to feel anything at all.

These feelings cannot be ordained but it is possible to create an atmosphere which does not prevent these emotions from arising, as unfortunately is all too often the case with a health care system geared to mere expediency. Nor is it my intention to propagate a certain way of endowing meaning, for it cannot be propagated in the same way for every person. My intention is only to illustrate that being sick inevitably poses final questions, that being sick indicates something transcendental, it leads a person to questions that transcend what concerns him in everyday life. Sickness precipitates a crisis, and a power can flow from the recognition of this crisis that can clear the mind and increase awareness. Modern medicine must not ignore this power arising from the crisis as has largely been the case until now because this power can have a beneficial effect if one only engages with the patient. To act in the capacity of a physician ultimately means to allow and even enable the patient's inner strength. To do this, the patient must learn to open himself to letting his inner healing power unfold. The physician and therapist can help him to see his having become sick as something asking to be actively overcome, something that gives him a mission so that he does not feel at the mercy of his sickness but even in sickness recognizes his resources for overcoming in his own way what is not desired. And this way only is an inner way, a spiritual way.

My intention in discussing the chance of inner healing power is simply to make it clear that what most patients need is an understanding person opposite them. They need assistance and support because especially in severe illnesses it can take time for people to find their way out the phase of helplessness and regain the ability to live their own life and reassert control over their life. That this can take a long time is due in part to the fact that they must first relate to their sickness in order to realize what the diagnosis means for them and the rest of their life. The diagnosis is not merely a fact. It involves ascribing meaning, and many physicians overlook this because they work in a health care system that is more concerned with objective and demonstrable facts than with hermeneutics. Yet they often neglect to consider that precisely the subjectivity that modern medicine seeks to methodically exclude is what is essential to learning to cope well with being sick.

If the physician only thinks in terms of target states and remains entrenched in this mindset, then he will only see the sick state as a deficient state that falls short of the target. This perspective not only leaves the patient alone but also squanders the potential that the every person has. Even and especially in the face of time that has become shorter, every person is fundamentally able to endow this time with meaning. He can fundamentally say yes to this time. In his distress, he only needs someone who helps him to say yes. Not to say yes only to the time that is coming and is becoming shorter, but also to say yes to himself and say yes to his life.

Therefore, we must not overlook the fact that even in the setting of incurable disease a person is capable of finding something like meaning in the awareness of a greater context. This assumes that we give him room to do so in our encounter with him and it assumes there is someone there who may be able to make him receptive for this new realm. In this way, every person can be healed without having to become healthy. He can be healed by overcoming the illness through his acceptance of it. This does not mean being healed by planning, by doing, or by expediently seizing control, but being healed by opening himself, by becoming attuned to the transcendental experiences that are not calculable or tangible. A human being can be healed even without the goal of physical healing depending on how he deals with his sickness, depending on how he integrates it into his life. The point is not to fall victim to our claims of being able to make the world and to recognize once again that in reality our happiness lies with us, not in our hands but in our inner attitude.

183

Notes

1 Christina Hölzle: "Psychosoziale Aspekte ungewollter Kinderlosigkeit," Statement before the expert hearing of the Enquete Commission on Law and Ethics in Modern Medicine on March 26, 2001, in Berlin. The appropriate statistics can be found in the annual reports at www.deutsches-ivf-register.de.

2 Peter Petersen: "Reproduktionsmedizin—Herausforderung an die ärztlich-wissenschaftliche Haltung der Menschwerdung," in: Udo Benzenhöfer, ed., Herausforderung Ethik in der Medizin. Frankfurt am Main: Peter Lang; 1994:81–98; here p. 90.

3 Martin Rhonheimer: "Die Instrumentalisierung menschlichen Lebens. Ethische Erwägungen zur In-vitro-Fertilisierung," in: Franz Bydlinski, ed. Fortpflanzungsmedizin und Lebensschutz. Innsbruck: Tyrolia; 1993: 41–64; here p. 53.

4 See "Die Last des unbekannten Vaters. Anonym gezeugte Kinder auf der Suche nach ihrer Herkunft," Radiofeuilleton Deutschlandradio of April 2, 2009. http://www.dradio.de/dkultur/sendungen/thema/944311/; see also "Auf der Suche nach der halben Herkunft," radio show 37 Grad of January 14, 2009. See also "Papa Mama Kind," Südkurier of December 3, 2009.

5 See Franz Böckle: "Biotechnik und Menschenwürde. Über die sittliche Bewertung extrakorporaler Befruchtung," Die neue Ordnung in Kirche, Staat, Gesellschaft, Kultur 1979;33:356–362.

6 Frank Nawroth: "Social Freezing—Pro und Contra," Der Gynäkologe 2013;9:648–652.

7 Martin Spiewak: "Die biologische Uhr anhalten," DIE ZEIT, Heft 39 of July 19, 2013.

8 See Deutsche Gesellschaft für Gynäkologie und Geburtshilfe, "Tiefgekühlte Eizellen—Möglichkeiten für spätere Schwangerschaften," published at: http://www.dggg.de/leitlinienstellungnahmen/stellungnahmen/.

9 Michael von Wolff: "Social Freezing: Sinn oder Unsinn?" Schweizerische Ärztezeitung 2013;94:393–395; here p. 395.

10 Claudia Bozzaro: "Ein Kind ja, aber erst irgendwann—Überlegungen zum Einsatz von Egg- und Ovarian-Tissue Freezing," in: Giovanni Maio, Tobias Eichinger, and Claudia Bozzaro, eds.. Kinderwunsch und Reproduktionsmedizin—Ethische Herausforderungen der technisierten Fortpflanzung. Freiburg: Karl Alber; 2013:233–249.

11 See Marianne Leuzinger-Bohleber, Eve-Marie Engels, John Tsiantis, eds., The Janus Face of Prenatal Diagnosis: A European Study Bridging Ethics, Psychoanalysis, and Medicine, London: Karnac Books; 2008.

12 Kirsten Wassermann and Anke Rohde: Pränataldiagnostik und psychosoziale Beratung. Aus der Praxis für die Praxis, Stuttgart: Schattauer;2009, p. 111.

13 Ibid., p. 29.

[14] From Monika Hey: Mein gläserner Bauch. Wie die Pränataldiagnostik unser Verhältnis zum Leben verändert, München: DVA;2012, appendix. See also Barbara Duden, Der Frauenleib als öffentlicher Ort, München: Luchterhand Verlag; 2007.

[15] ZEIT FORUM WISSENSCHAFT: "Per Gentest zum Wunschkind: Kommt bald die Schwangerschaft auf Vorbehalt?" Discussion on October 14, 2011, in Berlin-Brandenburgische Akademie der Wissenschaften Images.zeit.de/2011/43/ ZEIT-Forum-Fortpflanzungsmedizin. pdf (downloaded on January 6, 2014).

[16] Markus Dederich: Behinderung, Medizin, Ethik, Bad Heilbrunn/Obb.: Klinkhardt;2000, p. 264.

[17] Claudia Schumann: "Veränderungen in der gynäkologischen Praxis durch Pränataldiagnostik," BzgA, FORUM 1/2007, p. 341.

[18] "Ich wollte nicht abtreiben." Monika Hey im Gespräch mit Christiane Hoffmann. http://www.faz.net/aktuell/praenataldiagnostik-ich-wollte-nicht-abtreiben-11970680.html (downloaded on January 9, 2014).

[19] See Luc Boltanski: Soziologie der Abtreibung. Zur Lage des fötalen Lebens, Frankfurt am Main: Suhrkamp; 2007, Chap. IV.

[20] Irmgard Nippert, Heidemarie Neitzel: "Ethische und soziale Aspekte der Pränataldiagnostik. Überblick und Ergebnisse aus interdisziplinären empirischen Untersuchungen", Praxis der Kinderpsychologie und Kinderpsychiatrie 2007;56(Heft 5691):758–771, here p. 765.

[21] Maria Simon: "Danach. Die psychischen Folgen der Abtreibung," in: Paul Hoffacker, Benedikt Steinschulte, Paul-Johannes Fietz and Martina Brinsa, eds., Auf Leben und Tod. Abtreibung in der Diskussion, Bergisch-Gladbach: Lübbe;1991, p. 98.

[22] Maria Simon: Myriam, warum weinst Du? Psychische Folgen nach einer Abtreibung, Uznach: Uznach-Verlag; 1996:p. 106.

[23] Ibid.

[24] Marion Poensgen: Abschied von den unvergessenen Kindern. Frauen nach Schwangerschaftsabbruch und Adoptionsfreigabe, Freiburg: Lambertus Verlag; 1998.

[25] Simon: Myriam, warum weinst Du? loc. cit.

[26] Vgl. Hey: Mein gläserner Bauch, loc. cit.

[27] Lecture series "Lebenszeichen | Lebensentscheidung." Katja Baumgarten im Interview mit Sonja Toepfer. www.youtube.com/watch?v=qWSRHSmz9FQ (downloaded on January 9, 2014).

[28] From Hey: Mein gläserner Bauch, loc. cit., p. 174.

[29] Source: DAK (Deutschen Angestellten-Krankenkasse) press release of February 12, 2009 (www.presse.dak.de) Gesundheitsreport 2009. Analyse der Arbeitsunfähigkeit. Schwerpunktthema Doping am Arbeitsplatz. Hamburg: DAK, see http://www.dak.de/content/filesopen/Gesundheitsreport_2009.pdf. See also Stephan Schleim: Risiken und Nebenwirkungen der Enhancement-Debatte, in: SuchtMagazin 2/2010, and Jan-Christoph

Heilinger: Enhancement. Der Fortschritt der Wissenschaften und die Möglichkeit, Menschen zu 'verbessern', in: Dossier Bioethik der Bundeszentrale für politische Bildung (bpb): http://www.bpb.de/gesellschaft/umwelt/bioethik/160269/enhancement.

[30] The results of this study may be found in journal Pharmacotherapy: The Journal of Human Pharmacology and Drug Therapy January 2013:33/1:44–50.

[31] Source: MDKforum. Das Magazin der Medizinischen Dienste der Krankenversicherung, Heft 3/2010, Schwerpunktthema: "Neuroenhancement. Der Traum vom optimierten Gehirn."

[32] With respect to the medication Ritalin, see: Jörg Blech, Ulrike Demmer, Udo Ludwig, and Christoph Scheuermann: "Wow, was für ein Gefühl!" in: DER SPIEGEL, 44/2009, and Alexander Schwabe: "Ich bin ein Zombie, und ich lerne wie eine Maschine," in: DIE ZEIT of April 2, 2009; http://www.zeit.de/campus/2009/02/ ritalin (downloaded on January 18, 2014).

[33] Memorandum "Das optimierte Gehirn," Gehirn & Geist 2009;11:1 ff.

[34] "If couples (or single reproducers) have decided to have a child, and selection is possible, then they have a significant moral reason to select the child of the possible children they could have, whose life can be expected, in light of the relevant available information, to go best or at least not worse than any of the others." (Julian Savalescu and Guy Kahane: "The moral obligation to create children with the best Chance of the best life," Bioethics 2009;23/5:274–290, here p. 274.)

[35] Ilona Kickbusch: Die Gesundheitsgesellschaft. Megatrends der Gesundheit und deren Konsequenzen für Politik und Gesellschaft, Gamburg: Verlag für Gesundheitsförderung; 2006:69–71.

[36] Nach Don Nutbeam: "Health literacy as a public health goal: a challenge for contemporary health education and communication strategies into the 21st century," Health Promot Int September 2000;15(3):259–267.

[37] Bettina Schmidt: Eigenverantwortung haben immer die Anderen, Bern: Huber; 2008.

[38] Gernot Böhme: Leibsein als Aufgabe. Leibphilosophie in pragmatischer Hinsicht, Kusterdingen: Die graue Edition; 2003.

[39] Irmhild Harbach-Dietz: "Krebs und die Frage nach der Schuld," SIGNAL 4/2012, p. 28 ff.

[40] Helmut Dubiel: Tief im Hirn, München: Verlag Antje Kunstmann; 2006, p. 35.

[41] Giovanni Maio: Mittelpunkt Mensch–Ethik in der Medizin, Stuttgart: Schattauer; 2012.

[42] Klaus Steigleder: "Ethische Erwägungen zur Organtransplantation und zum Hirntod-kriterium," Bundesgesundheitsblatt 2008;51(8):850–856.

[43] See Sabine Müller: "Revival der Hirntod-Debatte. Funktionelle Bildgebung für die Hirntod-Diagnostik," Ethik in der Medizin 2010;22:5–17. See also: President's Council on Bioethics: Controversies in the determination of death. A White Paper. Washington, DC. http://www.bioethics.gov./reports/death/index. html.

[44] Ibid.

[45] Siehe Stefan Rehder: Grauzone Hirntod. Organspende verantworten, Augsburg: Sankt Ulrich Verlag; 2010.

[46] Fritz Blättner: Vom Sinn des Alters, Kiel: Hirt; 1957, p. 15.

[47] Romano Guardini: "Vom Altwerden," Arzt und Christ 1957;3:133–137, here p. 134.

[48] Thomas Rentsch: "Altern als Weg zu sich selbst," in: H. Blonski, ed., Ethik in Gerontologie und Altenpflege, Hagen: Kunz; 1997:93–104, here p. 283.

[49] Claudia Bozzaro: Das Leiden an der verrinnenden Zeit. Eine ethisch-philosophische Untersuchung zum Zusammenhang von Alter, Leid und Zeit am Beispiel der Anti-Aging-Medizin, Stuttgart: frommann-holzboog; 2013.

[50] Eva Birkenstock: "Altern und Selbsterhaltung. Zur Widergewinnung eines verdrängten Themas für die gegenwärtige Philosophie," in: Christian Iber und Romano Pocai, ed., Selbstbesinnung der philosophischen Moderne, Cuxhaven: Traude Junghans Verlag; 1998:193–208.

[51] Karlfried Graf von Dürckheim: "Der Sinn des Alters—Gereifte Menschlichkeit," in: E. Mendelssohn Bartholdy, ed., Souverän altern. Zur Psychologie des Alterns und des Alters, Zürich/Stuttgart: Classen; 1965:13–23, here p. 14.

[52] Odo Marquard: "Theoriefähigkeit des Alters," in: Ders., Philosophie des Stattdessen. Studien, Stuttgart: Reclam; 2000:135–139, here p. 137.

[53] Marquard: "Theoriefähigkeit des Alters," loc. cit., p. 137.

[54] Rentsch: "Altern als Weg zu sich selbst," loc. cit., p. 97.

[55] Ibid., p. 101.

[56] Hans-Martin Rieger: Altern anerkennen und gestalten. Ein Beitrag zu einer geronto-logischen Ethik, Leipzig; 2008:77.

[57] Rieger: "Altern anerkennen und gestalten," loc. cit., p. 103.

[58] Christian Mulia: "Altern als Werden zu sich selbst. Philosophische und theologische Anthropologie im Angesicht des Alters," in: M. Kumlehn, T. Klie, eds., Aging—Anti-Aging—Pro-Aging. Altersdiskurse in theologischer Deutung, Stuttgart: Kohlhammer; 2009:103–127.

[59] Rieger: "Altern anerkennen und gestalten," loc. cit.

[60] Source: Die Presse.com of June 18, 2012.

[61] See, for example, Brigitte Zypries: "Selbstbestimmung bis zum Ende," Frankfurter Rundschau of June 26, 2008, p. 12.

[62] Stephan Sahm: Sterbebegleitung und Patientenverfügung. Ärztliches Handeln an den Grenzen von Ethik und Recht, Frankfurt am Main: Campus [and others]; 2006.

[63] See the brochure of the German Federal Ministry of Justice on the living will, p. 36, http://www.bmj.bund.de/Publikationen/Patientenverfuegung_oe.html.

[64] Udo Reiter: "Mein Tod gehört mir," in: Süddeutsche Zeitung of December 21, 2013. See the response by Franz Müntefering: "Gefährliche Melodie," in: Süddeutsche Zeitung of January 3, 2014.

187

[65] Konrad Hilpert: "Der Begriff Spiritualität. Eine theologische Perspektive," in: Eckhard Frick, Traugott Roser, eds., Spiritualität und Medizin. Gemeinsame Sorge für den kranken Menschen, Stuttgart: Kohlhammer Verlag; 2009:18.

[66] Norbert A. Luyten: "Der heutige Mensch zwischen Wohlstand und Sinnerfüllung," in: Balthasar Staehelin, Silvio Jenny, Stephanos Geroulanos, eds., Engadiner Kollegium Vom Sinn und Wert des Lebens, Schaffhausen: Novalis Verlag; 1977:181.

[67] See Philippe Ariès: Geschichte des Todes. Translated from the French by HansHorst Henschen and Una Pfau, Darmstadt: Wissenschaftliche Buchgesellschaft; 1996.

[68] Paul Ricoeur: Lebendig bis in den Tod. Fragmente aus dem Nachlass, trans. and ed. by Alexander Chucholowski, Hamburg; 2011, p. 198.

[69] Ibid., p. 73 f.

Index